Social Work Practice in Nursing Homes

To my Colleague
Cathy. Best
wishes!
Julie Schleus

Also Available from Lyceum Books, Inc.

Social Work Practice in Nursing Homes
Creativity, Leadership, and Program Development

Julie Sahlins

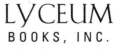

LYCEUM
BOOKS, INC.

Chicago, Illinois

© Lyceum Books, Inc., 2010

Published by

Lyceum Books, Inc.
5758 S. Blackstone Ave.
Chicago, Illinois 60637
773+643-1903 (fax)
773+643-1902 (phone)
lyceumbooks@lyceumbooks.com
http://www.lyceumbooks.com

6 5 4 3 2 1   10 11 12 13

ISBN 978-1-933478-73-9

Library of Congress Cataloging-in-Publication Data

Sahlins, Julie.
   Social work practice in nursing homes : creativity, leadership, and program development / Julie Sahlins.
       p. cm.
   ISBN 978-1-933478-73-9
   1. Medical social work—United States. 2. Social work with older people—United States. 3. Nursing homes—United States. I. Title.
   HV687.5.U5S25   2010
   362.61—dc22

                                                                2009006630

Manufactured in Canada.

To my family: Marshall and Barbara Sahlins, Peter, Elaine, Adam, Ramona, Lily, Gus, and Max, with love.

Contents

Preface

WHY WORK WITH THE ELDERLY, PARTICULARLY THE FRAIL ELDERLY WHO reside in nursing homes? For me, it is not about the money (although nursing homes provide a fairly decent salary in comparison with other areas of social work practice), nor of course is it about the prestige, which has in the past tended to be minimal but perhaps may increase as this population continues to grow. It is all about those intangible aspects of the work that make social workers tick. It is about helping a population that is truly at risk, physically, emotionally, and spiritually, to achieve a decent quality of life. It is about the opportunity to help people who are at a fascinating stage in life where, in our culture, we seek to make meaning of our existence. This life crisis often brings with it the gift of creativity, and I believe that it is an honor to be part of that process, by bearing witness as elders tell their stories and, in the telling, actually relive their experiences as they fashion them into a form that they can accept. Working closely with people at the last stage of their lives provides a unique opportunity to learn from the wisdom that they have accumulated over their lifetimes; to find out, in the end, what has really counted as a success; to draw important life lessons from their regrets; and to learn what, at the end of our days, truly matters. Working with the elderly can help the helper to accept the fact of death and to celebrate life, and the sheer joy of some of its ordinary rituals. In my mind, the question is not why work with the elderly, but why not?

In this book, I will share with you some of the ideas, constructs, and practices that I have developed (with the help of my clients, colleagues, and mentors) and found to be useful, ideas that were not part of my graduate school curriculum. It is my hope that the reader will benefit from this writer's struggles. After all, one does not become seasoned by blithely sailing through uneventful workdays. Instead, one becomes seasoned by learning (the hard way) from one's mistakes and errors. If I can spare some of you the trials and tribulations that accompanied the development of this conceptual framework, perhaps you will be able to more quickly reap the benefits of a practice that is mindful of anchoring our decision-making practices on the best possible use of our professional selves and then expanding upon these efforts in ways that have not yet been considered.

Recent thinking about organizational culture indicates that in the current climate of managed care, "standardization dominates the mood of most social service organizations" (Yan, 2008, p. 318). A nursing home setting is unique both in its challenges and in its opportunities. One of the greatest challenges is figuring out how the various components of the institutional system work, and work together, and how the social worker fits in. Several enormous benefits of this particular setting are the ability to work independently, for that work to have an impact on changing the mores and traditions in the setting, improving the quality of life for the residents, and influencing the development of a community that is responsive to their needs. The small social service departments in nursing homes are one area where standardization of roles may be expected, due to the existence of a corporate ethos, but this standardization is not set in stone. Here, it is possible for the lone social worker or tiny social work department to carve out a social service role within the institution and to use this role to transform the dominant culture. The existence of an interdisciplinary team of care professionals greatly helps to facilitate our ability to negotiate a social work identity (ibid.).

I strongly advocate for choosing an identity with its roots in the social work tradition of Jane Addams, whose myriad practical, cultural, and artistic programs were designed to meet the multidimensional needs of an impoverished community. Ms. Addams drew her inspiration from Toynbee Hall in England, the first settlement house, which provided comprehensive social services to a desperately struggling urban underclass based on the concept that "to help the poor, you must live with them and be available for all manner of daily needs and weekly crises" (Polikoff, 1999, pp. 53–54). Early community organizers such as Ms. Addams provide dynamic role models for the rich and fruitful professional identity that one can aspire to and even begin to approximate in our settings, with our "communities" of frail elders, where spiritual if not actual poverty exists in abundance. Almost paradoxically, the nursing home is a wonderful vantage point on which one can build an exciting and vital practice.

The ideas, constructs, and practices that I am referring to appear as themes throughout the book. A central concept is the importance of visualizing the entire facility in which we work as a sort of secondary client and the importance of engaging this "client" on many levels. Another important notion is that of maximizing our social work role by making full use of the wide spectrum of clinical skills that we have learned and continue to develop throughout our lives. A third emphasis is on using our professional judgment creatively to structure our role and activities so we can better address both the predictable and the unpredicted needs of our clients. Finally, another theme that is less prominent in the book but nonetheless important is for readers to keep in mind the need to take steps to monitor our efforts in order to maintain accountability for our work.

This book advocates for the social worker to seize the moment to make a difference. It is about the hand on the shoulder of a grieving family member or the supportive word to a stressed-out staff member. It is about seizing the opportunity to further the social work objective, whether that involves helping our clients to make social connections by organizing a cribbage game on the unit, having learned that two isolated residents love that game, or snapping a picture of a resident holding her great-grandson, surrounded by representatives from four generations of her family, and then presenting the picture to her to give to her daughter or have by her bedside, a tangible reminder of her identity outside of the nursing home. Finally, and perhaps most importantly, the reader will find that a core theme of the text has to do with programs. One social worker alone, or even a department of several, cannot meet the needs of a large caseload. Strategic program planning and implementation make sense in terms of increasing our effectiveness. The ability to make creative use of our professional selves is a tremendous potential source of career satisfaction.

This is a practical how-to manual, but by no means a cookbook. Please borrow my ideas, innovate on them, and make them your own. The aim of this book is to offer ideas for systemic interventions and program development that may help individual nursing home social workers (or those working in related settings) to fulfill their social work mandate while continuing to follow the highest standards of accepted practice.

In order to facilitate the reader's ability to follow the text, I will explain a little bit about how this volume unfolds. Chapter 1 provides the reader with a contextual understanding of the nursing home system and the role of the social worker in it. This overview of the system lays the foundation for discussion of various programs described in subsequent chapters, which represent social work interventions to serve the various needs of clients in this environment, based on the assessment of the social worker in collaboration with other interdisciplinary professionals. This programmatic approach, I believe, represents a disavowal of the twentieth-century trend toward strict endorsement of narrow theories and a movement toward the adoption of a variety of approaches based on research related to the importance of specific common factors—in particular, the curative aspect of therapeutic relationships in successful therapeutic outcomes, as opposed to the efficacy of any one particular orientation. Chapter 2 introduces the concept of using the construct of the facility as client and sets forth some very specific ways in which the social worker can apply this thinking to specific aspects of the traditional social work role in nursing homes. Chapter 3 discusses why life review is key to elders' well-being and sets forth the strategy of program development to address the de-emphasis on client individuality that exists in a medicalized setting. Reminiscence groups are specifically used to inaugurate this discussion because a focus on the residents and their memories is key to helping them reclaim their identities, as well as to promoting a focus on resident-centered care. Chapter 4 details some applications of art-making as a means of furthering the objectives of the life-review process. Chapters 5 through 7 describe ways that social workers can efficiently and effectively address the needs of their caseloads. The order in which the programs are discussed represents a movement from direct practice (groups for residents) toward more indirect methods of influencing various components of the nursing home system to effect culture change in the service of our clients. Nursing home staff are considered before family members because, from the point of view of the nursing home social worker, they are typically part of the system that more directly influences the residents' daily lives than do families, who are highly important to the residents' well-being but generally less visible to social workers who may not be present during the hours that they visit.

Chapter 8 is a culmination of this trend toward broader facility-based social work interventions that can help us modify our settings to become more humanistic. The notion of community mainly includes what exists within the building itself. Some of the objectives of this section are to encourage the social worker to strengthen a culture of caring within the facility and to foster the residents' sense of belonging to, as well as participation in, this community. Chapter 9 is situated after the lofty goals of the previous chapter to remind the reader that while we aspire to higher things, we still exist within the confines of our current settings, and that it is important to meet all of the more mundane aspects of our professional requirements. Chapter 10 is an acknowledgment of the existence of evidence-based practice as an increasingly important aspect of social work practice and discusses some steps that we can take to incorporate this reality into our work lives. Chapter 11 discusses various ways that social workers can maintain their professional identities and is specifically included at this point to emphasize that in order to maintain a strong social work department (even if it is only one person), it is crucial to remain connected with a professional network that can help to sustain us in this work. Chapter 12, "Final Thoughts," concludes the book and hands over to the reader the job of writing the next chapter, either metaphorically through programmatic interventions or perhaps in the next book on this subject.

Acknowledgments

TRULY, LIKE MANY ENDEAVORS, THIS BOOK IS THE WORK OF A NUMBER OF people and not solely of the author. I am indebted to and would like to thank, if inadequately, those who made this project possible. These include my program consultant, David A. Danforth, my friend and mentor, Ed Alessi, my astute readers, Marshall Sahlins, Bud Bynack, and Tom Meenaghan, and Peter Sahlins for his support and guidance at critical times (some of these roles overlap). I would also like to thank all of the nursing home residents whom I have had the privilege of knowing over the years, and in particular the veterans at the Chelsea Soldiers Home for all they have taught me.

Introduction

UNDOUBTEDLY, THE CLINICAL TRAINING THAT GRADUATE STUDENTS IN social work currently receive prepares them more specifically to meet the challenges of "real world" practice than did my own educational experience nearly twenty years ago. However, it seems inevitable that students' concurrent needs to learn how to provide quality clinical services while also mastering the tasks of negotiating the politics of an agency system and, at the same time, dealing with the intricacies of documentation cannot realistically be addressed within the relatively brief span of two years. The hopeful premise of this book, and books like it, is that it can help to bridge not one but two disparities. The first inevitable and understandable chasm is between the little clinical experience that we have upon graduation and what we must acquire, and the second, more mysterious, gap is that which exists between the knowledge we start with and other things that we haven't even considered yet (because we had no way of knowing ahead of time what they were and that we had to cope with them). While desiring to alert new social workers to the unexpected challenges and opportunities of our profession, at the same time it is my fervent wish to assist them in holding on tight to the idealistic principles that propelled us all into this profession, and perhaps as well to provide encouragement to more experienced folk like myself (because we can all use a reminder from time to time) to revisit the expectations, faith, and hope that brought us here, so that we can all remain vital in our work.

It is in this spirit that I share with you some of my own early experiences, ones which made resolving the apparent disconnect between my ideals and early clinical training and my experience of what happens "out there" a career-long quest. This introduction explores the culture shock that one fledgling social worker experienced when she found herself working in nursing homes, and how it set the stage for a versatile programmatic approach to caring for this particular specialized geriatric population.

FACING DILEMMAS

When I entered graduate school in social work school seventeen years ago as an older student, having already earned a master's degree in art education, following a bachelor's degree in painting, I had little training in the mental health field and a desire to help people and to improve their lives. My motivation to do so was probably born of the same mixture of unresolved conflicts and altruism that propels many new practitioners into the field of social work and that informs their first efforts at treatment. My professors taught me much, and my clients as much, if not more. I experienced healing in my clients and had some ideas about how a relationship infused with empathy, warmth, and genuineness might have contributed to a positive result (see Fischer, 1978).

Exactly how that healing had happened, however, was not entirely clear to me. It seemed and continues to seem that somehow, in my earnest listening to my clients, in my reflections on my work, in consultation with my endlessly patient, supportive, and humorous supervisor, and in my tentative suggestions about how to proceed, a spark was lit (not always, but often enough) that tended to kindle an excitement about the possibility of growth and change. No matter how much theory I have learned or will ever learn, it is a fact that defies explanation that there needs to be a synergy of this kind between client and clinician for healing to occur.

Synergy, beyond its general sense in ordinary discourse—that is, as mutually beneficial action—has two, more technical meanings. One is biological, the other theological. The biological definition is "the action of two or more substances, organs, or organisms to achieve an effect of which each is individually incapable." In theological terms, it is "the doctrine that regeneration is effected by a combination of human will and divine grace."

The social worker is the carrier of hope.

THE EDUCATION OF A SOCIAL WORKER

During my first-year fieldwork placement, back in the early '90s, I was given a total of eight clients at the D Street Mental Health Clinic, located in a gritty housing development and staffed by a committed staff of mental health professionals, including social workers, psychologists, mental health nurses, and a psychiatrist. The housing development may have been gritty, but the clinic was a warm and caring place. Inside the squat, unassuming brick building, plants and pictures created a homey environment. Clients and students alike were accepted, respected, and closely attended. A warm welcome and hot, albeit ersatz, coffee were always available to both clients and students.

In such a caring environment, healing was not unusual. I will never forget writing the last report for my final patient on the last day of my second year. My client, Mr. M, a gentleman in his early sixties who was in recovery from substance abuse, sought treatment for a stressful relationship with an alcoholic partner that threatened his own hard-won sobriety. Half-heartedly, Mr. M had attended NA meetings, battling an increasingly difficult war against his own addiction as the boyfriend's behaviors escalated to the point where he feared that he would show up at his place of work, sit on his desk, and humiliate him in front of his co-workers and boss.

A referral to AlAnon for Mr. M proved fruitful. He listened and took to heart the concept that he could not control the behavior of others, only his own. "Let the dishes pile up to the ceiling," he announced. "I'm not going to do them for him." As my client learned to detach himself emotionally from the situation, the partner's negative behaviors began to subside. Mr. M found new energy to pursue his interests in fixing up old cars and in gardening. My last process recordings were filled with his images of new growth as his flowers and vegetables prospered. On my final day at the clinic, he came running in the door, excitedly shouting for me to look at his newly renovated automobile. I think I will spend my career in pursuit of such flowering of life as I observed in this intervention, one of my first.

Only as a student, however, would I have the luxury of devoting so much time and attention to so few assigned cases. Although I wrangled a summer internship at the clinic, I eventually had to face leaving the womblike embrace of my first placement and of a very supportive and interesting second-year assignment at a child and family clinic. After that, encountering the real world of social work practice was a rude awakening. I felt completely unprepared. There was a lot that I hadn't learned in school.

This led me to ask what I had learned there. Seeking an answer to that question, I hauled out the box containing saved materials from my graduate school experience (I knew I had hung on to them for a reason). I wanted to compare what I learned in social work school with the challenges that I faced on the job after graduation. I am a nursing home social worker, and I wanted to try to identify what tools, if any, my graduate education had given me that functioned effectively in the environments in which I had been working.

The first paper on top of the pile, "Evaluation of Student Performance," was folded to the second page. I read:

Process and Technique
a. Competence in exploring and utilizing historical data; exploring affect and affectively charged information; dealing with resistance.
b. Ability to recognize and deal with transference and countertransference issues.
c. Skill in differential use of self.
d. Level of self-awareness.
e. Assessment of practice ability with individuals (adults, adolescents, and children), couples, families, and groups.

    f. Skill in work with larger systems, e.g., the organizations and community systems in which services are provided. Ability to identify and analyze gaps in the delivery system, recommended changes, etc.

    g. Performance in conferences, department or team meetings, staff meetings, etc. . . .

    h. Ability to evaluate own service. . . .

The list goes on. As I read these things, I realized that I had spent the last twelve years trying to adapt these principles, these evaluation criteria, to a practice that has less to do with social work than I could ever have imagined and more to do with nursing, and profit making, and a peculiar institutional culture.

The box of randomly saved papers was now spread across the floor. Hmmm. There were a lot of articles on clinical theory. And in this hoard of theoretical papers, I did in fact find three that, viewed retrospectively, from the point of view of my real-world experience in nursing home environments, actually do exemplify, although they do not summarize, a clinical approach to social work practice that provides an invaluable foundation to good clinical practice in the "real world" where that institutional culture prevails.

Example 1 "The Development of a Sense of Self" (Lichtenberg, 1975)

This is a discussion of theories about the development of a sense of self from infancy to early childhood. The author shows that "the sense of self can be seen as arising during an infantile stage as islands of experience that then, bit by bit, are formed into more ordered groupings of images. Bodily self-images, self-images in relation with objects seen as distinctly separate, and images of the grandiose self associated with idealized self-objects become blended experientially into a sense of self that has the quality of cohesion" (p. 482). A social worker who is familiar with developmental theories such as this is a social worker who is prepared to treat the selves with whom she has to deal as complex, evolved, and evolving entities, even those (or especially those) selves who are in the later years of their lives.

Example 2 "A Psychodynamic Approach to the Personality Disorders" (Stricker & Gold, 1988)

This paper stresses that, according to then-current psychodynamic theory, "unconscious mental processes exert significant motivational influence on behavior" and describes how character disorders can be linked to early developmental experiences through "psychic determinism" and "over determination." The authors note, cogently, that "a psychodynamically informed study of personality disorder utilizes these principals in a three-tiered approach to diagnosis and treatment. The first, and most evident, tier includes the observation of symptoms, behavior patterns, and eliciting situations that identify the individual as suffering from a personality disorder. The second tier is focused on the present and over determined meanings of the ongoing overt behaviors. . . . The third tier of understanding is aimed at identifying the developmental/historical antecedents that determine the behavior" (Stricker & Gold, 1988, p. 351). The authors conclude that this "three-tiered psychodynamic conceptualization of personality disorders . . . offers clinicians enhanced opportunity for understanding the complexity of etiology and current functioning of personality disorder, and adds considerably to focused selection of treatment techniques" (p. 358). A social worker who is familiar with developmental theories and has been trained to approach cases using "a number of intrapsychic and systemic viewpoints" (to quote the Advanced Clinical Practice syllabus) is a social worker who is prepared to understand her clients' dilemmas on many levels, especially when those clients bring with them a lifetime's worth of developmental/historical antecedents and experiences.

Example 3 "The Capacity to Use the Object" (Newman, 1984)

This article compares the two major theories of Melanie Klein and Heinz Kohut in their understanding of what constitutes object usage by a patient and concludes (in part) that "the analyst's activity through listening or offering an interpretation or identifying a feeling state must communicate the possibility of more positive relationships with others than those that were established in infancy" (p. 168). A social worker capable of listening to and interpreting the client's verbalizations on several levels can facilitate healing in a number of ways, not the least of which is applying object-relations theory in innovative ways to the very real task of easing the transition of nursing home residents from the lives that they have known to the life that they must live in their new home.

In short, I realized, in social work, as in my previous experience in the field of visual art, theory can be a foundation for practice. A comparison could be made between a graduate student learning clinical concepts in order to practice social work competently and an art student learning art theory in order to be able to paint proficiently. Like an artist, a social worker is taught a variety of skills and techniques by accomplished and experienced teachers, and just as an artist becomes adept at communicating meaning through her art, we as social workers use our skills to help clients find meaning in their lives. A strong theoretical foundation provides us with many tools that we can adapt as the situation requires, in accordance with the clients' needs and our own idiosyncratic tendencies or styles.

Take, for example, a new resident's concerns about her admission to the nursing home. The resident arrives by stretcher, accompanied by two emergency medical technicians and trailed by her frazzled daughter. They are escorted without fanfare to an available room by a busy nurse, who tells them she will be back shortly to do her assessment. Before coming to the nursing home, the resident was in the hospital. Perhaps she fell at home during a cardiac incident. Perhaps her husband died quite recently. It has been decided that this woman will need nursing home care.

A social worker is perfectly positioned to intervene in this situation, and her training in clinical theory provides the basis for and guides this intervention. This is a life crisis involving a major life change for the client and her family. Moreover, it is clear that there are many psychosocial issues here, most of them involving loss (loss of spouse, loss of health and independence, loss of her role in the family and role in the community). It is also clear that there is a benefit to having a trained social worker interview this resident and her family to assess the client's mental status, mood and coping skills, and developmental needs and to provide support to facilitate her adjustment.

The social worker can develop a rapport with this resident and her daughter, listen and empathize with their current situations, find out the salient facts about the resident's condition and her coping, as well as the coping of her daughter and family. She can listen to and reflect upon their feelings and in doing so provide a context for healing to occur. She can explore the resident's life history, including occupation, family relationships, and interests. In doing so, she is not only validating the new resident's identity and making sure that other staff are aware of her individuality, she is increasing the new resident's self-esteem and ability to cope with the major life change that nursing home admission entails.

If we apply object relations theory to the situation of a newly admitted nursing home resident who is struggling with feelings of anger and resentment, we realize that we can strive to use our relationship with the client to support the positive feelings that she has about the significant others (past and present) in her life and help her to preserve her current relationships, despite the disruption caused by the placement.

However, there is more to a real-world situation than clinical considerations. Let's say that the social worker is actually available at this time, on this day, to meet with this new resident, and that she actually does get a chance to do her assessment, provide support and comfort to the resident and family member, and develop a care plan that facilitates the new resident's adjustment. But to what is the resident adjusting? An institutional setting, a rigid routine, a focus on her physical needs that will be attended to by an overworked staff, and separation from her family and her community, with only organized activities such as bingo, movies, and van rides to relieve the monotony. And unlike a social work intern, an actual social worker in a nursing home has many more than eight or ten cases, none of them at scheduled times and none whose situations initially appear to have much to do with clinical theory.

As a new nursing home social worker, I realized quickly that my job was divided into fifty-minute hours. Indeed, the overt agenda with which I was presented involved a daunting series of tasks defined by the nursing home agency and the administrator. I struggled with confusion about how to remain true to social work principles while fulfilling all of the stated requirements of the job in a corporate and medically oriented environment where there was no support to be had and no one spoke my language. Instead, the nursing home has its own language. It's a language that a social worker needs to hear and to learn.

A nursing home social worker is expected to complete certain sections—sections AA, AB and AC, AD, A, possibly B and E, F, and sometimes P, Q, and R—of the Minimum Data Set for each of the residents upon admission and on a quarterly basis, at minimum, and more often in certain situations, for example, when the resident has been hospitalized. The social worker must complete notes in the residents' charts at least quarterly (more often in certain cases), the content of which is not standardized. She must note any hospitalizations, changes in the residents' medical conditions, responses to stressors, coping, level of orientation, level of family involvement and of residents' socialization, behavioral issues, if any, and social service plans and goals. Of note is the fact that a common and expected social work goal is to visit with each resident one-on-one at least weekly. A little math will tell you that with more than eighty residents, this is unlikely, if not impossible.

In addition to the above responsibilities, there are meetings and crisis interventions with upset residents and family members. Moreover, the social worker generally has such assigned tasks as informing elderly residents and their families when a room change is deemed necessary by the administration. In facilities where a lot of short-term rehabilitation occurs, frequent room changes are common. It is well known that such change is disruptive and disorienting for an elderly population. Yet, as a nursing home social worker, I have been informed by more than one administrator that a "strong" social worker can "convince" residents and families to move with ease and efficiency. Finally, the social worker is expected to be the residents' advocate. This is a role fraught with conflicts of interest because the social worker's livelihood depends on maintaining the good will of her employer.

A typical day in the life of a nursing home social worker embodies these conflicts and stresses. In it, the tensions between the agenda of the social worker and those of the nursing home management and the administrator are clear.

It's 9:00 a.m., time for the morning meeting. Department heads hurry up to the fourth floor for a "stand-up" meeting with the administrator. The meetings are supposed to be short—about fifteen minutes—but they usually last about forty-five. Each department head is supposed to say what he or she is doing that day. A new resident is coming for rehab. Treatment: broken hip. The social worker is required to make calls to families to make bed changes to accommodate the new arrival. She knows that neither the current resident nor her family will want the resident to move. She's been in that bed for years—and she has a window. . . .

10:00 a.m. Interdisciplinary care plan meeting. The Minimum Data Set (MDS) has been completed, each discipline having done the required sections. Now four residents and their families are scheduled to meet with the staff— that is, with the unit nurse, physical therapist, occupational therapist, nutritionist, and social worker. The MDS coordinator times the meetings with an egg timer, and no family member is allowed more than fifteen minutes. We read them the care plan and ask if there are any questions. The family member complains about lost laundry. This complaint is cut short by the care plan coordinator. Make an appointment with the social worker, she suggests.

10:30 a.m. The social worker goes off to complete various tasks. Predictably, the resident with the window bed and her daughter are very upset. They refuse to move. The administrator is displeased.

11:00 a.m. Medicare meeting. We find out that two residents are ready to be discharged tomorrow. The social worker must contact the families and make transportation arrangements, ensure that an oxygen tank is delivered (promptly) to one home, make referrals to the Visiting Nurse Association, Meals on Wheels, and adult day care, and make sure that a three-page referral is in place.

12:00 p.m. The social worker is about to go to lunch when she is paged. Mr. X wants to leave against medical advice. He has no family, and his mental status is questionable. She convinces him to stay one more day. . . .

1:00 p.m. The social worker is paged again and asked to give a tour.

2:00 p.m. Time to try to catch up on paperwork while eating lunch. There are three phone calls to return. There are five MDS assessments due tomorrow, five quarterly assessments, plus notes, and forms to fill out for the welfare department to extend a resident's benefits. Plus three new residents came in yesterday, and their psychosocial assessments need to be completed. . . .

3:00 p.m. The social worker is paged. Mrs. Y. has been refusing to take a shower—again.

4:00 p.m. The exhausted social worker finally gets to visit a few of her residents.

4:15 p.m. Drop everything! "The state" (the Department of Public Health) is here on an abuse evaluation. (This does not happen every day, we hope.)

The nursing home is based on a hospital model of care, and medical decisions there are often driven by financial considerations (the proverbial bottom line). The MDS mentioned above is a tool used for reimbursement of Medicare and Medicaid payment to the facilities. It behooves the facility fiscally to maximize its Medicare payments. Engaging in rehabilitation treatment is one way to do this— short-term admissions to the facility for the purpose of physical and occupational therapy and skilled nursing care. Thus, the focus is on "filling the beds" with short-term residents, giving them as much treatment for the acuity of their illness as insurance allows, then discharging them back into the community when the limit of their insurance reimbursement is reached. As a result of the focus on rehabilitation treatment, the needs of long-term-care residents are generally neglected by the overextended social worker because, in general, the ratio of residents to social worker is around eighty or ninety to one and much of her time is taken up making sure that discharge deadlines are met as a priority.

Amid these conflicting priorities, there is pressure on the social worker to adopt completely the priorities of the facility and its administration. It is hard to remember that we entered the field of social work because we wanted to help people. It is also hard to remember that once upon a time, we were taught about object-relations theory and the psychology of the self. We use our interpersonal skills to de-escalate crises, but whether we are trying to empower our clients or to manage them for the purposes of the institution can become murky.

If, as we are encouraged to do, we have joined our professional organization, we can turn to the National Association of Social Workers and their code of ethics. As a new nursing home social worker, in the privacy of my office, between telephone calls and pages, I picked up my copy of the National Association of Social Workers Code of Ethics and read it.

The preamble states that "the primary mission of the social work profession is to enhance human well-being and help meet the basic human needs of all people, with particular attention to the needs and empowerment of people who are vulnerable, oppressed, and living in poverty. A historic and defining feature of social work is the profession's focus on individual well-being in a social context and the well-being of society. Fundamental to social work is attention to the environmental forces that create, contribute to, and address problems in living" (National Association of Social Workers, 1999).

Read in the context of the daily life of a nursing home, this document raised more questions than it answered. How can the social worker empower the nursing home resident? How can we address their "problems in living"? How can the powerful tools of clinical theory be put to effective use in such a setting? How can the synergy between social worker, client, and staff that I experienced during my training occur in real-world settings that sometimes appear to discourage it? How can I, the only social worker in the nursing home, continue to carry hope, when hope is in such short supply?

I believe that part of the answer is to consider the entire nursing home as a client—albeit a resistant one. With the nursing home as a whole as our client, we must use our skills to make an alliance, to develop a shared language, identify common goals, and find a way to implement them. Later chapters show how, in practice, we can begin to do this.

Chapter 1

The Social Worker in the Nursing Home System

THE WORLD OF LONG-TERM CARE RESIDENTS IS A VERY CLOISTERED ONE, wherein their lives are very much determined by the daily realities of the institution. If we come to work in such a setting, eventually, inevitably, we ourselves become a part of this type of system and learn to perform, for better or for worse, an integral role in its functioning. It is therefore doubly important for our clients that, as their advocates, we try to understand as much about the dynamics of our facilities as we possibly can. What follows in this chapter is a brief history and analysis of the American nursing home (and a little bit about the development of our own profession). This information is intended to provide background material for the reader to consider when formulating an understanding of how she fits into the culture of her setting and a model of the social dynamics that exist in this particular system.

TAKING STOCK

If we accept a job as a nursing home social worker, we are stepping not only into a medical care setting for the frail elderly, carefully decorated in tastefully coordinated colors reminiscent of a hotel lobby or corporate boardroom (mauve and green are common), but into a situation steeped in historical influences that we may not be aware of, but whose effects we will soon inevitably detect in the policies and procedures of the institution, as well as in the ritualized ways in which the staff members relate to the patients, their families, and to each other—the very culture of the nursing home. The new social worker can quite unknowingly allow herself to be socialized into the culture that exists in her building and thus be co-opted into accepting the role that others assign to her, a role that does not always make use of her skills and training. Alternatively, she can try to understand the system she has entered and use this unique opportunity to work strategically as part of its small, enclosed world to create a vital person-centered community for her clients within the walls of the institution.

Presently, a small but significant number of people, approximately 1.4 million, live in approximately 16,000 nursing homes across the country. More than half of these nursing home residents are over eighty-five years old, and most are female. Two-thirds of these individuals have more than one chronic medical condition, and six in ten residents have both medical diagnoses and related cognitive impairments (Weiner, Freiman, Brown, & RTI International, 2007). Thus, although there are exceptions, of course, such as recent admissions of younger mentally ill and/or homeless individuals, as well as patients who are admitted for rehabilitation following health crises, then discharged to more independent settings, in general, when we talk about nursing home residents, we are talking about one of the most fragile and vulnerable segments of our population and, also, not coincidently, a disenfranchised group with little social prestige or status: medically compromised elders without many financial resources or a network of support from an extended family.

The facilities that house these people are mostly proprietary. Sixty-seven percent of nursing homes are privately owned (Gabriel, 2000). More than half of all nursing home facilities are part of large corporate chains (Harrington, Carrillo, and Woleslagle Blank, 2007). This situation has not been conducive to positive outcomes in terms of meeting the residents' individualized needs, as illustrated in a *New York Times* exposé (Duhigg, 2007). This article documented decreased staffing patterns, along with attendant decreases in the ability of residents to function and increased depression, accompanied by many lapses in regulatory oversight following corporate takeovers.

Nursing homes run by large corporations attempt to marry a profit motivation with care for frail elders. Here are some statements to that effect from their own Web sites: "We can maximize profitability only if we provide quality care" (Sun Healthcare Corporation, n.d.). "Satisfy customers with quality care and compassion" (Beverly Living Centers, n.d.). And "We will be the recognized leader in clinical quality and customer satisfaction in every market we serve" (Genesis Healthcare, n.d.). This peculiar mix of capitalism and compassion for elders and their families *as consumers* says much about our ambivalence as a society about this segment of our population. We feel a moral obligation to take care of our elders, but since doing so ourselves is not a priority in our youth-oriented culture, we allow the market forces to dictate the terms of that care.

In recent times, the Culture Change Movement, united under the Pioneer Network, an umbrella term for several grassroots organizations involving long-term care providers and advocates, have begun to challenge the way that nursing homes do business and advocate for a more humanistic model of care. These organizations and others have developed paradigms of person-centered care that feature practices such as grouping residents in neighborhoods instead of wards, granting more autonomy and status to direct caregivers, and incorporating more homelike features into the residents' daily routines, such as the presence of pets, plants, and visiting children (Fagan, 2003).

Indeed, the current model of nursing home care in these corporations and in smaller companies needs critical examination as an acceptable way to care for the old and sick. The existing institutional system is a deficit-based one, built on the assumption that its residents are not only a problem for society, but people with problems (Brody, 1974). In addition, the medical model that is used to address these people's "problems" in many ways reinforces this negative focus. Care plans are developed from an assessment of the residents' medical, emotional, and psychosocial difficulties. Only incidentally do nursing homes emphasize the clients' strengths and support networks or attempt to build on these.

How has this situation come to pass? The institutional model of care to which nursing homes tend to conform was shaped by many sociological and economic forces. In this chapter, I will explore the some of the influences that have shaped today's nursing homes.

THE ORIGINS OF CORPORATE NURSING HOME CULTURE

One author who has examined the early history of the modern-day custodial institution is David Rothman. Rothman (1971) traces the development of long-term care in America from the colonial period to the late nineteenth century. He argues that whereas in the colonial era, dependent persons were treated at home or in settings that resembled private dwellings, in the spirit of enlightened reform, institutions such as prisons, psychiatric hospitals, orphanages, and almshouses were developed by a newly industrialized society to meet the needs of "deviants and dependants. Unfortunately, these institutions did not fulfill their promise as model environments for efficient and effective rehabilitation. They lapsed into poorly run and unregulated holding areas for persons unwanted in society at large and were eventually taken over by private industry. However, their legacy has endured.

Rothman shows that, before the Civil War period, colonial Americans, like their English predecessors, believed that the existence of the poor, the sick, and other dependent individuals (such as the frail elderly) was "inevitable and God given." Thus, at this time there was only a limited social stigma attached to being poor or needy. Communities were close knit, and it was recognized that a reversal of fortune could happen to anyone. Assistance to those in need was administered on the local level and tied to the unit of the family as the provider of care whenever possible. In colonial days, Rothman (1971) notes, institutions for the care of the unfortunate were modeled both architecturally and functionally on the ordinary household: "The almshouse patterned itself upon the family, following this model as closely as possible. The structure, typically located well within town boundaries, lacked both a distinctive architecture and special administrative procedures. Some settlements did not bother to construct a poorhouse; instead they purchased a local farmhouse and used it without altering the room divisions" (p. 42). Colonial Americans saw no need to distinguish or separate themselves physically from the poor and the needy—except perhaps from the "outsiders" who immigrated from other countries or towns and were perceived as threats to the economic resources of the community.

All of this changed in the Jacksonian period, when the more ordered society of earlier times became less structured and more fluid due to industrialization and immigration. Instead of viewing the poor as neighbors in need, early-nineteenth-century Americans saw them as victims of inadequate family life, subject to the temptations of vice and corruption inherent in an industrial society. Reformers sought to remedy this situation by constructing facilities that, in structure and administration, ended up looking much like the impersonal factories of this era.

An 1866 report of the Commonwealth of Massachusetts Board of State Charities revealed the new stigma associated with this remedy when it noted that "these institutions have a double function: they serve as residences and receptacles." The new institutions were built to promote social order and structure at the same time that they separated the inhabitants from the general population. Prisons tried to separate the inmates from the negative influences of their peers by incarcerating them in solitary cells and enforcing silence during communal meals. Mental hospitals endorsed a strict therapeutic routine and were designed to administer this efficiently and effectively. Poorhouses or almshouses, with their associated workhouses, while also intended to be well-ordered places, did not have as clear a mandate as these other institutions. They served as dumping grounds for the very young, the old, the sick, and others on the margins of society.

Thus, instead of addressing society's ills by providing the disenfranchised (including the frail elderly) with orderly living situations that were separated from the community at large, these "enlightened" institutions by and large degenerated into situations of quasi-incarceration—poorly regulated, at that, and neglectful in their administration. Nevertheless, their legacy has endured.

What has also endured, unfortunately, besides the factorylike structure of our present-day institutions, are the negative effects on an individual's personal and social identity of living in a "total institution" (Goffman, 1961). Irving Goffman describes the process by which institutionalization breaks down a person's identity in terms that are chillingly relevant to today's nursing home residents—

although he was speaking of inmates in prisons and patients in mental hospitals. "The inmate finds certain roles are lost to him by virtue of the barrier that separates him from the outside world," writes Goffman (p. 16).

The process of entering a nursing home typically brings other kinds of loss and mortification as well. We generally find staff employing what are called admission procedures, such as taking a life history, photographing, weighing, fingerprinting, assigning numbers, searching, listing personal possessions for storage, issuing institutional clothing, instructing as to rules, and assigning to quarters. Admission procedures might better be called "trimming" or "programming" because in thus being squared away the new arrival lets himself be shaped and coded into an object that can be fed into the administrative machinery of the establishment, to be worked on smoothly by routine operation (Goffman, 1961).

The resemblance between the modern nursing home and this institutional model has occurred to more than one critic. Sheldon Tobin (2003) notes: "Nursing homes fit Goffman's criteria for 'total institutions' where residents, patients, inmates or religious orders are handled in 'batches'" (p. 54). Tobin identifies the goal of this particular institution in a way that parallels Rothman's description of the function of the Jacksonian poorhouse: "Whereas most total institutions handle inhabitants primarily for the purpose of resocialization, nursing homes do so for efficiency" (ibid.). He concludes, as I have, that "while saving money, efficiency usually conflicts with humanistic goals" (ibid.).

To add to this unfortunate situation, as we know, the forces that shaped the contemporary nursing home have also included the private for-profit industry. After the "enlightened" reform that saw the development of modern institutions, including almshouses, fail as a government enterprise, and once federal funds became available for the care of the elderly, individual entrepreneurs saw on opportunity for investment and developed this interest into large corporate organizations.

Kaffenberger (2001), in a discussion of the economic influences shaping the current nursing home, shows that understanding the history of corporate involvement is a simple case of following the money. Reforms in the Progressive Era in the early twentieth century, Kaffenberger notes, led to the passage of old-age assistance pensions for the elderly. These funds enabled an increasing number of elderly persons to live in private and public lodgings and boarding homes, often owned and run by nurses. Shortly after this, in 1935, President Roosevelt signed the Social Security Act, which provided funds to seniors but would not pay for public long-term care facilities such as almshouses. This, in turn, encouraged the development of even more board-and-care establishments, rest homes, and nursing homes to meet the demands of the senior market. Eventually, the

Federal Housing Authority began to finance both public and private nursing homes. The industry expanded astronomically, particularly in the private sector, between the 1930s and the 1960s. Finally, in 1965, the Medicaid and Medicare Acts were passed, again increasing the incentive for industry to take advantage of the market, because Medicaid, in particular, paid for long-term nursing home care.

This "financial feeding frenzy" led to both pecuniary fraud and resident abuse. In response, the Omnibus Budget Reconciliation Act, which was passed in 1987, contained legislation regulating nursing homes—the 1987 Nursing Home Reform Act. This act had the salutary effect of creating some basic standards of care and dignity in the nursing home. These included "residents' rights, minimum nursing staffing, an interdisciplinary team approach for evaluating and care planning, measurable goals, creation of a uniform resident assessment instrument (RAI) focused on functionality and self-care, development of the minimum data set (MDS) for comprehensive care planning and outcomes justification and monitoring of physical and chemical restraints, training for nursing assistants, and a revised quality of care survey that was resident-focused" (Tobin, 2003, p. 58). The regulations also institutionalized the need for a full-time social worker.

ENTER THE SOCIAL WORKER

In 1987, when nursing homes were mandated to employ social workers to meet the psychosocial needs of the residents, they received a group of individuals trained in a helping profession that was, at the time, approximately one hundred years old. These people, primarily women, were skilled in casework, group work, social advocacy, and knowledge of human psychic functioning.

We can trace this legacy of social work in America to the period following the Civil War. The war, with its devastating effect on veterans and families—together with the poor working conditions, cyclical depressions, and unemployment spawned by the escalating process of industrialization—gave rise to a need for social action and social reform. Women who had become involved in wartime philanthropy took leadership roles in the organized charity movement that followed. The Charity Organization Movement ultimately developed into the field of social work—which remains predominantly a female profession (Trattner, 1994).

The initial mission of the Charity Organization Movement was to help the poor in a scientific way. Using "friendly visitors," generally of the upper classes, the project involved gathering information on the causes of poverty and dependency. This led to the existence of professional schools of social work with a legacy of advocacy and social change. In particular, it stimulated Mary Richmond to develop the formal technique called social casework. In 1917, she wrote *Social Diagnosis*, the first casework textbook in the emergent discipline.

In the 1920s, social work aligned itself with the psychoanalytic movement, with its emphasis on the individual at the expense of a focus on the poor and the causes of social injustice (Woodruff, 1971). While this alignment has imbued the profession with knowledge of the human psyche and has helped to increase its acceptance as a valid profession in the eyes of the medical community and the larger world, in some ways, it has narrowed its focus. What may have been overlooked as the social work profession has matured is some of the earlier idealism, notably the kind that went into the exciting and highly successful settlement house movement of the late 1880s.

The settlement house movement was similar to the Charity Organization Movement in that both relied on volunteers and shared the goal of improving the condition of the poor through personal relationships. Moreover, both movements emphasized scientific inquiry and investigation. Both also tended to be somewhat idealistic, developing out of a worldview defined by spiritual and even religious qualities (Trattner, 1994).

Best exemplified by the famous Hull House of Chicago, founded by Jane Addams and Ellen Starr, the philosophy of the settlement house movement was based on the "Three R's"—"Relationship, Research, and Reform." Settlement workers went to live in poor neighborhoods, developed relationships with the neighborhood residents, and brought about social change by developing programs to solve local problems. Settlement House workers sought to be inclusive of other cultures and to value ethnic identity. They helped to develop vibrant local communities, rich with art and culture. They engaged in political advocacy. In many ways, I feel that they are the models to which social workers should still aspire to this day.

However, for better or for worse, social work took a different course when the settlement house movement declined in the early twentieth century, in part due to its unpopular stance against World War I, and also due to the increasing professionalization of social work, which involved aligning itself with the field of psychoanalysis and shifting its focus away from the urban poor to a more affluent population in an effort to gain social recognition (Trattner, 1994). While the benefits of the professionalization of social work are many, I feel certain that the lessons of this period in our history have much to teach us about revitalizing the spirit of the profession of social work.

THE SOCIAL WORKER AND THE NURSING HOME TODAY

Initially a potentially unwelcome guest in the nursing home, with an agenda different from that of the nurses or the administration, the social worker of the 1980s may have at times found herself feeling powerless and overwhelmed in a confusing and peculiar culture—a situation that still applies today. The alliance between the social worker and her facility remains a tenuous one. The social worker must continuously assert her role, or she may find all of her time taken up ordering eyeglasses, possibly even engraving dentures, and doing other tasks unrelated to social work at the request of the administration or the nurses.

The social worker must walk the line between the use of creative program development in the tradition of Jane Addams to meet the specific needs of her population and compliance with the current version of the OBRA regulations, MDS 2.0 (soon to be 3.0), and care planning and documentation. Instead of simply accepting the facility's definition of her role, the social worker needs to find a way to make this role her own, based on the mandates of her profession, her clinical judgment, and a belief in her own creative spirit. The support of the professional organization, the National Association of Social Workers, with its *Standards of Nursing Home Practice* (see, for example, National Association of Social Workers, Massachusetts Chapter, 1996), is important in this regard. So, however, are strategies and tactics that will enable the social worker in a nursing home to define that role and act effectively within it. In the chapters that follow, I hope to provide such strategies and tactics and to enable nursing home social workers to act and work professionally within the constraints of the nursing home environment.

Presently, there are a number of reform initiatives of interest to the nursing home social worker. Some focus on institutional change, such as the Pioneer Movement and the programs that it endorses (Baker, 2007). The effort here is to replace the medical model of nursing home care with a paradigm based on community—to create a resident-centered life in which the nursing home is indeed a "home." These ideas and some of the results that their advocates have achieved are truly remarkable. The efforts of these groups are important and necessary. However, in practice, it is not always possible for social workers to adopt these reforms. A major reason is that these initiatives emphasize the need for institutional change to be embraced by the administration and introduced into the facility by leaders who are invested in its principles. The social worker is not in a position to influence her administration directly to do this.

Since it is unlikely that nursing home social workers can convince administrators to embrace immediate reform, in the meantime we must go about this process indirectly, quietly using our clinical skills at relationship building to take a leadership role in the task of transforming what is now primarily medically focused care to a more holistic way of thinking about the minds, bodies, and spirits of our residents.

Chapter 2

New Approaches to Nursing Home Social Work

ONE OF OUR GREATEST ASSETS AS SOCIAL WORKERS IS OUR ABILITY TO see the forest, as well as the trees. Our understanding of the larger system of the nursing home and our role in it is a perspective that the other professionals in the building may not necessarily have, and it gives us the very special ability to strategize to effect positive change within those systems on behalf of our clients. We are then said to be working with a system as a "secondary client," which we usually do at the same time that we are helping our clients on an intrapsychic level and sometimes at the same time as we help them negotiate other systems in their lives (such as their family system) in order to help them to reclaim their identities and achieve some level of mastery over their environment. When working with secondary clients, as with primary clients, the first step in the process is always for us to try to understand our client at the same time as we are developing a working alliance with them. In the case of the nursing home as client, we need to develop multiple alliances with multiple aspects of the system. Only then can we truly be effective.

As we saw in the last chapter, because of the way in which the nursing home system evolved, the role of the social worker in today's nursing homes is in some ways laced with contradictions. The modern nursing home has its roots in government-sponsored care of the sick, the poor, and the elderly who lack family support networks and in a medical model of care based on the hospital. And because most nursing homes today are corporately owned, in practice, decisions are generally made outside the facility by administrators who are often in a different state and who favor a cookie-cutter approach to almost everything from menus and decor to nursing policy and procedures. Additionally, these unseen executives tend to micromanage individual facility administrators with an eye toward profitability and toward maintaining a uniform corporate culture across all of their buildings. Financial profit is tied to a high rate of bed occupancy in the nursing home, as well as to extracting the maximum amount of Medicare funding for rehabilitation services and acute nursing care. Thus, focusing on these items is a huge priority for corporate managers, and therefore individual administrators in individual nursing homes consider these things to be of paramount importance, which is at odds with the social work agenda.

The traditional role of the individual social worker in this system is complex and varies from place to place, but some factors can be generalized. For instance, the social worker is considered part of the "support staff." Nursing is the biggest department, and the most powerful, because nursing care drives reimbursement, and the nurses make up the bulk of the administration of each facility. Moreover, the social worker is not a direct money maker and thus in some ways she falls below the members of other support departments in importance, such as the rehab team (composed of physical and occupational therapists), that bring in revenue. Thus, in terms of the social hierarchy, the social worker is fairly low on the totem pole.

Regarding the formal chain of command, the social work director usually reports to the administrator, as do the other department heads, such as the directors of nursing, rehabilitation services, dietary services, activities, housekeeping, and maintenance. It should be noted that there are situations in which the director of nursing may have greater authority than the administrator in making medical decisions. As for the social worker, she may have one or two other helpers, but most often no more than that. And as we have seen, although the social work standards developed by the Massachusetts National Association of Social Workers Nursing Home Committee and adopted by the full NASW mandate that at least one full-time social worker be on staff for every eighty beds, this is a lower ratio than what typically exists in the real world. Likewise, at least nominally, the role of the social work director is that of a middle manager like that of other department heads, in practice, when the department heads meet briefly each morning to discuss issues of concern, the social work director is well advised, in this forum and others, to seek permission from the more influential director of nursing when proposing potentially controversial suggestions and in general to seek consensus from all department heads that may be affected by any particular social work intervention. Such is life low on the totem pole.

THE SOCIAL WORKER AND THE MDS

Life low on the totem pole means a life of paperwork. The practice of social work always involves an inevitable amount of paperwork, and in the case of nursing home practitioners, this is tied to a state and federally mandated assessment that is necessary for both funding and regulatory compliance: the MDS (Minimum Data Set), which identifies residents' problems and tracks their medical status, functional abilities, and emotional concerns. While use of the MDS has helped to eliminate the worst cases of abuse and neglect, it and the other nursing home regulations instituted with the 1987 Nursing Home Reform Act not only have encouraged an emphasis on medical outcomes, rather than on a process of caregiving that supports quality of life, they also have led to a focus on the documentation of official procedures, rather than hands-on interpersonal interactions with residents (McLean, 2007).

While there is no particular regulation stating who fills out what sections in the MDS, social workers, depending on the requirements of their facility, may be responsible for any or all of several sections having to do with demographic information, residents' prior customary routines, mood and behavior patterns, psychosocial well-being, and discharge potential (Beaulieu, 2002). This means that the social worker is at risk for adopting the impersonal values that, as a result of the MDS, permeate the customs and mores of the nursing home, because the institution places a great deal of emphasis on its timely completion at the expense of the social worker knowing her residents and being aware of their personal characteristics, feelings, and desires. I recommend that the social worker be diligent in filling out her sections of the MDS while keeping in mind that there is a difference between social work values and the priorities of the institution in this instance.

However, life low on the totem pole doesn't prevent you from keeping your eyes fixed on higher goals. The real issue here is how to reach those goals. Ultimately, I believe, the answer lies in realizing that the nursing home residents, the staff and administration, the corporate owners, and the social worker herself exist within a single biopsychosocial system. It lies in serving the interests of the residents by treating the facility itself, as a whole, as her client.

When we cognitively reframe the situation in this way, our task now becomes the development of a working therapeutic alliance with this client around shared goals (David Danforth, personal conversation, June, 13, 2006). The principle underlying all such interventions is that in a closed system such as the nursing home, the basic biopsychosocial assessments that you learned in graduate school can be combined with a thorough systems assessment and implemented through the development of relationships not just with your primary clients, but with the entire extended client system. Thus, we can strategically effect systems change in the service of all our clients and facilitate the fit between the residents and their environment.

THE SOCIAL WORKER'S ROLE WITH THE FACILITY AS CLIENT

It is the systematic nature of the nursing home that accounts simultaneously for the ability of the social worker to affect conditions positively, the inevitability of conflicts within the system, and the efficacy that someone trained in social work brings to the resolution of those conflicts. Systems theory evolved from the efforts of the behavioral sciences to incorporate insights from biology, psychology, and the social sciences into an understanding of human behavior (Hammond, 2003). Although it has presently fallen out of vogue in some quarters, systems theory is invaluable in understanding group dynamics in terms of the feedback, self-regulation, homeostasis, and adaptation of various biopsychosocial systems.

For example, one component of the nursing home system on which the social worker can have a direct, positive effect is the interdisciplinary team. This influence can be out of proportion to her institutional standing, and the reason for this is because the system also functions in informal, noninstitutional ways. The interdisciplinary team convenes weekly for individual residents' care-plan meetings on each unit. This team is composed of all of the clinical staff responsible for the particular resident's care. The composition of the team varies slightly from one nursing unit to another. It includes the nurse unit manager, the clinical assessment nurse or MDS coordinator, the nutritionist, and representatives from the rehabilitation, recreation, and social services departments, as well as the resident and his or her responsible party, most often a family member. The MDS coordinator or the unit manager most often coordinates these meetings and is ultimately responsible for clinical decisions made in them. However, each team member is expected to contribute his or her professional expertise. As a result of the informal status acquired in the group, the social worker can be quite influential in advocating for the resident's psychosocial needs. This, incidentally, points out the extreme importance of the social worker knowing each resident, including his or her history, past identity, interests, and current functioning, so that she can contribute suggestions for meaningful personalized interventions.

CONFLICTING EXPECTATIONS OF THE SOCIAL WORKER

In addition to advocating for residents' psychosocial needs in weekly care-plan meetings, a major role of the social worker in the nursing home is to advocate for the residents' rights as guaranteed by the federal 1987 Nursing Home Reform Act. (Resident rights include the guarantee of dignity, choice, and self-determination.)[1] A copy of these rights is given to the resident (or family, if the resident is not competent) on admission to the nursing home and, according to each state's department of public health, is supposed to be reviewed annually with the resident. Moreover, the social worker is expected to assist residents and families with adjustment to the facility, as well as with significant events affecting the residents, and to resolve crises involving residents and families. Each of these social work functions can, in fact, present a conflict of interest for a social worker employed by a long-term care facility. Many conflicts, however, can be dealt with by creatively applying the skills that social work teaches. And each conflict reveals a little more about the nature of the nursing home as a biopsychosocial system.

Advocacy

Although nursing homes are mandated to have social workers, and their own mandate is to advocate for the residents, in reality, the social worker's ability to perform this function is mitigated by her need to maintain an allegiance with the administrator, facility, and corporation that provide her with a job and pay her salary. At times, this represents a conflict of interest for the social worker, who must try to balance the needs of the facility and her loyalty to the nursing home with the needs of residents and families. As noted in the Introduction, a good example of such a conflict of interest is when the social worker is directed by the administration to facilitate room changes. Changes of any kind are notoriously difficult for the elderly, and it is said that the psychological effect of a room change on a frail older person is as stressful as that of a younger person having to move to another city. Change and stress can negatively affect an elder's coping and even physical well-being, sometimes precipitating a downward spiral of depression, inactivity, and poor nutrition that can be devastating and even lead to death. (This dynamic is also of great concern when a senior is initially admitted into a nursing home.) Nevertheless, the exigencies of admitting short-term patients for the purpose of rehabilitation and discharge and the necessity of accommodating these individuals if they are unable to return to their former living situations sometimes requires that long-term nursing home residents be "asked" to relocate from a skilled nursing unit (where rehabilitation or skilled nursing can be reimbursed by Medicare A) to a long-term care floor. In these cases, it is the social worker who is responsible for presenting the mandatory 48-hour written notice to the resident and family, but this notice can be officially waived and the resident moved immediately if the resident and family agree to the transfer. Here, of course, the needs of the resident and those of the facility are in complete opposition, and it is up to the social worker to weigh and balance all of the factors involved, including a realistic assessment of her influence with the administration, the unique needs of and the anticipated effect of the proposed move on the individual resident, the resident's and the resident's family's relationship with the staff and the facility, and the existence of alternative solutions to the problem in order to decide if advocating for the resident to stay in her present room is a battle the social worker can strategically afford to fight while still maintaining a working alliance with administration, or, if not, how she can best help to mitigate any negative effects of the move.

All of this serves to point out, again, that the influence of the social worker in the nursing home environment is particularly effective when it is an indirect one. As opposed to having formal power and authority, the social worker's ability to effect change is based primarily on her alliances with individuals and groups within the facility. Fittingly, this is what social workers are trained to do: develop alliances. Thus, the social work function in a nursing home (and probably in other types of settings, as well) can be conceptualized as an untraditional one where basic casework skills such as the establishment and maintenance of therapeutic relationships are applied to various aspects of the social work setting itself in the service of the residents—the primary clients.

Adjustment

The priorities of the nursing home do not necessarily include making individual accommodations for each resident. Instead, residents typically are expected to "adjust" and fit into the routines of the nursing home, be compliant with care, and attend generic recreation programs such as bingo and van rides. The facility generally expects the social worker to help residents "grieve" their losses of health and independence and to reassure them of the benefit of being cared for at the nursing home, where they can be visited by their families, make new friends, and enjoy staying as active as possible. Sometimes, general support and reassurance are enough to ensure the residents' relative well-being. Often, however, they are insufficient to address the really drastic insults that the loss of their home and a move to the nursing home represents to a person's self-esteem and very sense of selfhood on many levels. Once again, the interests of the institution and the professional imperatives of the social worker are at odds. Once again, the social worker's training provides a way to deal with the conflict. And once again, by playing an effective role within the system of the nursing home, the social worker serves the needs of both the residents and the facility itself as clients.

A very important service that social workers can perform for their clients entering the nursing home is to bolster the residents' sense of identity by taking a really good social history, focusing prominently on the basics—ethnicity, family of origin, education, primary life role (occupation or perhaps role of mother in a family), military service, if applicable, adult family roles and relationships, relationships with children, pets, extended family, friends, hobbies and interests, including clubs and organizations. A resident's understanding of her medical condition and feelings about the health losses that necessitated the need for nursing home care are also crucial pieces of information in understanding who this person is. Finally, the social worker needs to understand the resident's expectations about the admission (long term versus short term) and feelings about having been admitted, such as feelings of abandonment by their family, that can be anticipated as a normal response to placement but can be devastating both to residents and to families in terms of maintaining their relationships. If all of this sounds fairly obvious, it is, but too often, in practice, the social history is neglected by nursing home social workers and a brief check-off form takes the place of a reasonable evaluation of the client's biopsychosocial situation.

Once she has obtained a very good history, the social worker can share this information effectively, informing the interdisciplinary team as well as the nursing assistants about the resident's roles and accomplishments. She also can encourage the family to bring in pictures for the resident's bulletin boards, which can serve as both transitional objects for the residents and conversation starters for caregivers to begin get to know their charges as individual human beings. The social worker can work with the activities director to provide individualized programs for new residents, possibly including unique interventions developed specifically to help them maintain some aspects of their former identities. Some examples might be obtaining legal journals for a former lawyer to peruse (even if she can no longer understand them fully), helping a former shutterbug to take pictures with an inexpensive camera, working with the activities department to provide yarn and a crochet hook for someone who loved to crochet, or helping them to do a new craft, if their manual dexterity has changed. Recently, I completed an assessment on a new resident, John, a man in his 50s with an unfortunate degenerative illness that left his mind fairly intact, but his body uncooperative. Finding out that one of his favorite pastimes was playing cribbage, I mentioned to another cribbage player, Garry, that he might have a partner. Garry was interested. That afternoon, a call to his nurse sent him wheeling down in his chair to John's unit, cribbage board in tow. The two found an empty table and were still playing when I left the ward an hour later.

The social worker can provide even more extensive interventions by developing explicit programs based on common interests that residents on her caseload share—a topic that I'll address at length in a later chapter. The point here is that when it comes to facilitating the adjustment of the new resident, seen properly, the interests and procedures of the institution and the social worker advocating for the residents are not ultimately at odds after all. The adjustment always is mutual, because it occurs within a larger system. In fact, the facility must make individual accommodations for each resident if the nursing home is truly going to be anything resembling a home where residents fit into routines, are compliant, and participate in the life of the home with a sense of belonging that is so necessary to us all as social beings. The social work assessment here is key.

Conflict and Crisis Resolution

Finally, no system can survive if it is taxed with sustained, unresolved conflicts. Conflict resolution is a role that is generally agreed to fall squarely into the purview of social workers. These conflicts can take many forms, from disputes between roommates over whether the window should be open or closed to family complaints about their loved one's care.

Some of these situations are straightforward and do not represent a particular conflict of interest to the social worker, but others are more complex and problematic. For instance, in the case where a family is critical of the nursing home care, many factors may be at issue, including the family's guilt about placing their loved one in a facility, their unrealistic expectations of the institution, the resident's distress about the loss of his or her health and independence, the way the staff may approach and interact with the resident and/or family, as well as possible lapses in the quality of care delivery on the part of the staff. To add to these concerns, because most institutions are run for a profit, and even those that nominally are not face tremendous financial pressures in the current economic climate, the administration and staff may react to such family complaints with an instinctive "us versus them" mentality, almost automatically perceiving the family as "difficult," overly demanding, and antagonistic to the smooth functioning of the institution.

In any case, it is up to the social worker to help resolve these often messy situations and to promote a solution that is acceptable to all parties. In this instance, a major dilemma that the social worker faces is her mandate to advocate for her client and, by extension, her client's family support network, while at the same time coping with the necessity of maintaining an allegiance to her employers and a working relationship with them.

One key to resolving this conundrum is simply to be aware of the existence of this conflict of interest. Listening attentively to both sides will help the social worker to adjust her strategy when advocating for the resident and family and to· reframe the problem in a way that reflects goals shared by both parties—the well-being of the resident. Then, if the social worker is able convey to all parties that their needs have been heard by her and to convince them to hear each other, she will have gone a long way toward resolving the problem. In fact, at this point, surprisingly, with or without social work facilitation, staff members often are able rather quickly to develop their own appropriate interventions.

THE FACILITY AS CLIENT

As the conflicts of interest inherent in conflict resolution between the facility and its resident suggest, in a closed system such as the nursing home, it is important that the social worker consider the system where she works as a secondary client. Indeed, the importance of doing so cannot be overestimated. Without a thoughtful analysis of the dynamics of the setting and a conscious awareness of the various ways that these can affect both her and her primary clients, the residents, the social worker cannot effectively advocate for those clients, help them adjust to the facility, or resolve issues within the system. All of this, by the way, very nicely fits in with the social work role described in the NASW code of ethics, as described in the preamble:

> Social workers promote social justice and social change with and on behalf of clients. "Clients" is used inclusively to refer to individuals, families, groups, organizations, and communities. Social workers are sensitive to cultural and ethnic diversity and strive to end discrimination, oppression, poverty, and other forms of social injustice. These activities may be in the form of direct practice, community organizing, supervision, consultation, administration, advocacy, social and political action, policy development and implementation, education, and research and evaluation. Social workers seek to enhance the capacity of people to address their own needs. Social workers also seek to promote the responsiveness of organizations, communities, and other social institutions to individuals' needs and social problems. (National Association of Social Workers, 1999)

The paradigm of the facility as client is not one that is often articulated as part of the social work role in nursing homes, but it is especially relevant in closed systems such as long-term care settings. In traditional social work, workers attempt to view the larger picture of the client's "ecosystem": the family and the formal and informal support networks that make up the client's reality, as well as the stressors that affect their world. In the nursing home, the residents' lives are so tied up with their dependence on the staff and so highly structured by the routines of the facility that their ecosystem largely becomes the nursing home, with the family diminishing in importance in relation to this huge entity. The residents are affected, for better or for worse, by any changes in that system.

Figure 1 shows a diagram of the system. Thick and thin arrows throughout the diagram denote the impact of various parts of the system on each other. The resident (small circle) is affected (arrow) by the nursing home (big circle). The thicker arrows indicate a strong impact of the nursing home on the resident, whereas thinner arrows indicate a weaker impact of the resident on the nursing home. Similarly, the resident and the family have reciprocal effects on each other (in this case, both strong ones, as indicated by the thick arrows). The nursing home itself is shown as containing many smaller units designated as "administration," "nursing," "activities," "dietary," "rehabilitation," and "social service," all affecting each other. The nursing home is affected and modestly affects in turn the even bigger corporation.

Figure 1. Diagram illustrating some of the relationships between various parts of the nursing home system (in three-dimensional space).

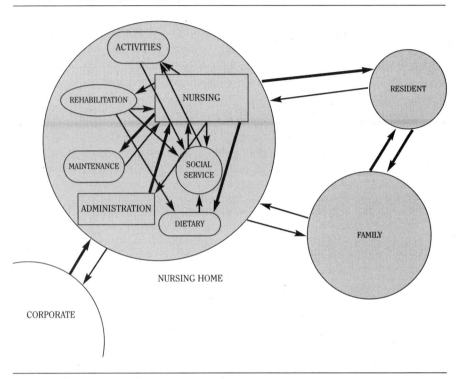

Whether advocating for her clients individually or as a group, helping them adjust to the facility, or assisting with problem resolution, the social worker derives a great deal of her potential power from her ability to formulate a biopsychosocial assessment and to see the large picture that makes it clear how an impact on any one aspect of the system may affect the client, for better or for worse. Moreover, a change in the nature of the relationship between the various aspects of the system (the arrows) will also affect the client. Because the social worker is also a part of the biopsychosocial system, an acute awareness of her role in that system is necessary if she is to use herself effectively. Being part of the system can be exceptionally rewarding because, due to relationships with the clients and with others in the system, the social worker can frequently plan and execute individualized interventions very effectively.

The concept of the social worker developing and maintaining fluid, workable alliances on many levels and with many aspects of the facility is an extension of the social worker's ability to do so with secondary clients in the primary client's ecosystem. However, at present, in schools of social work, developing and using working relationships with many aspects of the nursing home facility—considering the facility as a client—is not a focus of professional training. Yet without this subtle reframing of the social worker's role, we are vulnerable to having the system define our job for us in ways that may not benefit either our clients or ourselves.

Considering the nursing home as a client defines the way we approach every aspect of the system. Instead of reacting angrily or with some other unchecked emotion to the actions or comments of a coworker or administrator who might not understand or value the benefit of social work, we can more constructively respond by considering this action to be an artifact of a (possibly resistant) component of the system as client, a component that must be understood and thoughtfully managed—as should any countertransference thoughts that we might have. In lieu of such dysfunctional responses as avoidance of engagement or treating the client in an adversarial manner, we will now show the facility as client the same respect that we have for our primary clients and "meet them where they are," whether this happens to correspond to our viewpoint or not. Thus, if a nurse manager's priority is the residents' physical well-being, but the manager does not see the necessity of accommodating "overly demanding" family members, it is our responsibility to bond with the nurse around our shared concern for the residents' medical needs and to work with them to help them to recognize that preserving the residents' relationships with their families will affect their psychological state and thus, ultimately, their health.

Defining the social worker's role vis-à-vis the facility in this way and developing the ability to be both an outsider taking the long view and an insider negotiating solutions through the use of relationships also enables us to be assertive in our role, because it shifts the focus from an adversarial standoff between individuals to one of cooperative problem resolution within a larger system. This more neutral, professional stance will ultimately gain the nursing home social worker increased respect from others in the system. Joining with others by empathizing with their position and treating them as equals does not always work; in this the social worker does not always prevail, but this stance helps to defray some of the conflicting expectations that I have described as being inherent in the social work role. This reframing of the situation gives us the ability to empower ourselves to accomplish more and also may help us to gain a both a sense of control and more actual influence than we might otherwise have had in performing our job.

REFRAMING: STARTING TO WORK WITH THE FACILITY AS CLIENT

The facility can often be a challenging and resistant client. The social worker's first task is to establish a trusting, mutual relationship with that client. To that end, small successes in achieving an alliance are important and should be valued. Over time, many small, positive interactions based on shared goals can develop into a powerful force for change. A basic step in this process is to make daily rounds on the units, visiting with residents and stopping to check in with nurses and nursing assistants, also checking in with the nurse manager about how a particular resident is doing, demonstrating to them that a social worker can contribute to this patient's well-being, letting them know that she actually performs a useful function the daily life of the facility and is not merely an uninvolved person with an ill-defined role who can be made useful by running errands that nobody else wants to do.

The facility's trust can be earned in many ways: by providing psychosocial information about the residents to the staff, by spending a little time sitting with a dying patient, by helping to initiate hospice services, by working with families to structure pleasant visits, or by ensuring that relatives bring in pictures of their family to serve as transitional objects for that resident and to remind them (and the staff) of their identity. The nursing home social worker can demonstrate to the medical staff through her actions and the positive results in the residents' moods and affects what her job is, how she can benefit the patient, and how her involvement can lead to better patient outcomes. This will create a synergism of positive energy that the social worker can build on by working collaboratively with other interdisciplinary staff members. For instance, our shared interest in developing programs for the facility led me to collaborate with the nurse manager of our Alzheimer's unit to work with the staff developer to send us, along with several staff members on that unit, to the annual state Alzheimer's association conference to learn and teach others new approaches to the treatment of this population.

At the same time as she is developing relationships with residents and staff on all levels and working on developing new programs, it is imperative that the social worker be up to date with her progress notes—a minimum standard of competency as a professional—and that she "does her part" by completing her sections of the MDS in a timely manner. (Not doing so is upsetting to the MDS coordinators who are responsible for the completion of these documents.) Many nursing home social workers say that this alone takes up all of their time, and certainly it can. However, the better you know your residents, the less time it takes. Moreover, there may be a certain avoidance on the part of social workers (and other nursing home staff) of truly getting involved in the lives of their residents. Getting close to our frail, elderly residents leaves us open to the pain of losing them. Burying ourselves in paperwork is one way of dealing with the sad reality that many of our clients will die in the not too distant future.

However, this situation usually leads to job dissatisfaction. Moreover, this coping strategy is a disservice to our clients, particularly to the long-term residents who need us to be present both physically (as much as possible) and emotionally to help make a difference in whether they truly live during their remaining time in what is probably their final home or merely exist, waiting to die. And in serving our primary clients in this way, we also serve the facility as client by making it the kind of place that it should be.

FOCUSING ON SPECIFIC ASPECTS OF THE CLIENT SYSTEM

There are many ways that the social worker can work with her secondary client, the facility itself, to enhance the residents' quality of life. These include: reinforcing the identity of the interdisciplinary team by validating the contributions of team members and helping to ensure that decisions about residents' care are made by the team as a unit, helping to increase staff sensitivity to residents' needs and feelings, and establishing and maintaining a family council (see chapter 7). Many of these systemic interventions can be done on an individual as-needed basis as part of the social worker's day. Others can be most efficiently accomplished by establishing groups or programs, which is why the development of programs is such an important though currently underused clinical resource.

Strategizing: Finding a Middle Ground

Inevitably, there will be times that you disagree with the care-plan team. When, where, and how to negotiate a solution are all things that vary from institution to institution. These things must be learned by each social worker through a careful analysis of the particular setting and by constant reevaluation of the system based on observation, new information, and trial and error in making such decisions. This boils down to clinical judgment, a skill that comes with training, practice, and experience. Because such judgment is developed and not something with which we are born, it is important for new social workers and social workers new to nursing home practice to seek mentors, group supervision, and other forms of support and ongoing education.

A situation that I experienced in my practice helps to illustrate clinical decision making in a closed system and how to find a balance between client advocacy and maintaining a relationship with the facility as secondary client.

Case study

Joe, a seventy-year-old married veteran and former owner of a small laundry business, had a diagnosis of chronic obstructive pulmonary disease and depression. He was a smoker. Joe had four daughters, one of whom is a heroin addict who had recently relapsed. He resided in a barracks-type ward in a veterans' facility. Within a year's time, many deaths occurred on this unit. Most of these deaths occurred in the bed next to his, and although one bed change was made, per his request, all of the new residents who were placed next to or near him died. He had witnessed the most recent death. Joe was in treatment with the facility's contracted psychiatric service and was seen for weekly counseling and medication management. He was on an antidepressant (Wellbutrin), and the dose had been increased recently due to his increased symptoms of depression and irritability.

As part of his care plan, Joe's nurse manager had been working with him to educate him about the consequences of smoking for his medical condition. He stated that he wished to quit smoking, yet refused assistance and treatment to help him with this goal. The staff were frustrated with his noncompliance. Joe perceived his nurse as rigid and controlling and treated her accordingly. When yet another veteran was placed in the newly vacant bed next to his, he became even more angry with his nurse and was verbally and physically aggressive toward the new resident. A meeting was held where Joe expressed that he felt that terminal patients were deliberately placed next to him. The staff empathized with Joe's distress about the deaths, but ultimately dismissed his concerns, basically stating that deaths occur on all the units and that he would have to get used to them. This only exacerbated his anger and aggression. He was subsequently sent to the local emergency room as a psychiatric emergency but returned several hours later, having been deemed to be not a risk to himself or others.

At the next brief morning meeting, as the unit social worker, I said that I did not feel that, as a group, we had listened closely to our patient. I noted that he had been trying to verbalize his distress about the deaths in beds adjoining his and other stressors and his wish to move for some time, and while we had tried to address his stress and depression, we had not been responsive to his desire to move. I added that this was his right and stressed our shared mandate of client advocacy.

In deliberately speaking in terms of what "we" had done, I allied myself with the facility and phrased my advocacy for the resident in terms of a mutually important goal. This last piece was the clincher for the administration, and they strategized to identify the best unit for Joe. He was moved the next day. He adjusted very well to his new location, and his symptoms of anger, aggression, and depression improved immediately and remained stable.

This example shows what may not have been a perfect clinical social work intervention. Perhaps the patient could have been moved before his frustration escalated; these deaths all occurred next to or near him and probably led him to believe that he might be next. In addition, the social worker could have worked to explore the client's fears and in doing so could have helped to resolve his anxiety. However, this is a real example, and the intervention did have a positive outcome. It demonstrates the social worker working strategically within her relationship with the facility as client to advocate for a resident. This story also illustrates the trial-and-error component of the social worker's lifelong learning curve. As a professional, this situation led me to be more sensitive to the effect of a death on the other residents, to be more vigilant in assessing this effect, and to be more active in assessing the residents' fears and facilitating their grieving. In the process of doing this, I also work with the staff to increase their awareness and responsiveness to this issue.

CHOOSING YOUR BATTLES

However effective it may be to treat the facility as a client, there is a difference between serving the needs of that client and complicity with the nursing home system in all things. Our duty in these matters supersedes our allegiance to the facility, and in the unfortunate situation where we must choose between the two, we must choose uphold our ethical responsibilities.

We must adhere first to our code of ethics, and to the regulations of our board of licensure as a top priority. If you are asked to do something by your facility that appears to be in serious violation of these principles, you must not compromise yourself by this action. Your license might be at risk. If you need help, get help: call your supervisor, your consultant, your NASW Board of Ethics, or a trusted colleague for advice. Recently, in Massachusetts, a social worker was reported to the Social Work Board of Registration for an ethical violation and also for not complying with a regulation requiring that she receive supervision, something for which her facility did not pay. This demonstrates that we cannot rely on our nursing home administration's judgment alone in meeting our professional duties. In fact, we must not only be aware of nursing home regulations pertaining to social services, but familiar with our code of ethics and up to date on licensure regulations.

There are times, then, when it is necessary for the social worker to take a stand on the ground of the profession's fundamental values. Our priorities in doing so can be summarized as ensuring the physical safety of residents, ensuring their psychosocial well-being, and maximizing their independence and safeguarding the exercise of their rights.

Resident Safety

It is our duty to intervene if we feel that a resident is at risk from harm or injury to self or others. We may come to the conclusion that there is such a risk after completing an assessment of the client and his or her situation. For example, we must act, as in the case of Joe, the angry and aggressive resident discussed above, if the resident poses a danger to the physical safety of himself or others. Moreover, in the case of residents with dementia, agreements reached with them to alter their behavior are likely to be meaningless, and we need to rely on our clinical judgment to protect the patient and others. It is crucial to document that we have done all that we reasonably could to ensure patient safety. This includes discussing the case (or making sure that the case has been discussed) with the upper levels of nursing management, as well as with the physician, who has the final word in addressing the situation. Ideally, we should also refer the case (or make sure that the case has been referred) to a psychiatrist, who is recognized as an authority on clinical judgments but whose opinion is considered to be only a recommendation to the physician. If the nursing management does not wish the case to be referred to a psychiatrist, we should include this fact in our progress note.

Of course, if at all possible, we should not leave a scene where resident safety is at issue until the situation is addressed, and we should document the result in our notes. We should document as well the fact that we have taken all reasonable measures ourselves to ensure patient safety, including removing the patient's access to any items that could be misused and recommending to nursing that measures such as ten-minute checks or one-on-one supervision be put into place if we feel these to be necessary and nursing has not implemented such measures already. The bottom line: document, document, document!

Ensuring the Resident's Psychosocial Well-Being

We should prioritize our need to intervene more directly in cases where the team disagrees with us in terms of minimizing any potential risk of psychological injury to the client. An example of a high-priority intervention would be advocating to avoid changing a resident's unit to accommodate the needs of the facility if that resident is grieving a recent significant loss, such as the death of a child, or experiencing stress, such as a new diagnosis of cancer. Such a situation requires the presence of familiar staff to provide the resident with a sense of continuity.

Maximizing the Residents' Independence and the Exercise of Their Rights

We should take a stand in situations where the client's independence and rights are at risk of being seriously curtailed. A fairly common example of a time when the social worker may need to advocate strongly for a resident's independence and rights is when a competent client wishes to go home but the care-plan team discourages or even ignores this wish in their desire to "protect" the resident.

LIMITS OF THE PARADIGM

If we lived in a perfect world, all nursing home social workers would have small caseloads and lots of time to attend to them, with no unnecessary meetings or paperwork, so that we could practice the client-focused interventions we were taught in social work school. Other members of the staff would always respect (and even usually agree with) our opinions, and we would be able to represent all the residents' needs, because their holistic well-being would be the medical staff's and administration's main agenda.

Unfortunately, in the real world where we live and work, this is not often the case. At times, because they have a different frame of reference and as a result of external pressures, others in the nursing home system may seem difficult to engage. Some of the social worker's suggestions may go unheeded, and her efforts may appear to be unappreciated. It is hard not to take all of this personally, and the tendency is to internalize these difficulties, rather than to respond thoughtfully to them. The truth is that while we cannot directly affect many aspects of our institutional surroundings, at least we can reframe them for ourselves in a way that allows us keep functioning as client advocates and agents of cultural change. By treating an impasse with our the client system similarly to the way we would work with a resistant client, we can find ways to address many difficult situations creatively.

Working within this new construct does not ensure that the social worker will always be effective in controlling certain aspects of the environment. Nor does it mean that the social worker will be immune from becoming caught up in the interpersonal dynamics or politics of the workplace. While mistakes (our own and others'), upsets, and roadblocks can be disheartening, we can always learn from them and refine our understanding of the system. The rewards of working in this way are deep and meaningful connections with our residents and their families, the support of the colleagues whom we have successfully engaged in collaborative professional relationships, and, most importantly, the ability to make a difference for our clients. Another case study illustrates the effectiveness of developing relationships within the system as a whole in effecting change.

Case study

Walter, a former army air force pilot, took a last stand. When the housekeepers came to pack up his roommate Steven's belongings (Steven was in the hospital, but still alive), Walter stopped them. He said, "Wait a minute. I'm in charge here, and I've been watching his stuff for him. The only people who will clean it out are his family. See, I'm keeping it for him." He showed me a tiny replica of the World War II destroyer on which that Steven had served, which he had carefully stored in Steven's locker.

I marveled that Walter had taken a position that I hadn't—that I couldn't have taken. After all, how could I tell the nursing home to lose money on a bed that could be filled? Yet imagine Steven's daughter's devastation to see her father's area packed up, stripped bare. I thanked Walter. He was eighty-eight years old. He was considered a notoriously "difficult" and demanding resident. Yet at that moment, Walter was not a nursing home resident. He was a soldier who wasn't about to leave another soldier behind. The best part about it is that the administration let him. The workers left the room empty-handed and were not asked to return. I guess we were all humbled in the face of his humanity.

How can we preserve such humanity in an institution? By encouraging friendships like Walter and Steven's to flourish. By cultivating them. Dispassionate, inflexible rules aren't conquered by a lone social worker taking a stand. They are conquered by the power of relationships.

Note

1. These rights are detailed on the Medicare Web site www.medicare.gov. See also the online publication, Guide to Choosing a Nursing Home, at http://www.medicare.gov/Publications/Search/Results.asp?PubID=02174&Type=PubID&Language=English.

Chapter 3

Reminiscence and Reminiscence Groups

THE IDEA OF CONDUCTING SUPPORT GROUPS AND DEVELOPING OTHER types of programs to meet the psychosocial needs of nursing home residents is not presently mandated in most current job descriptions for nursing home social workers, nor is inventiveness such as this in social work practice particularly encouraged in schools of social work. However, in fact, therapeutic groups are an important way that social workers can maximize their own resources, and, moreover, this treatment modality can have a significant effect on the lives and well-being of our clients. Group interventions are an efficient, effective way to address residents' psychosocial and life-stage-related concerns, and they also effectively

Figure 2. Group co-leader listens as a resident reminisces during a group session.

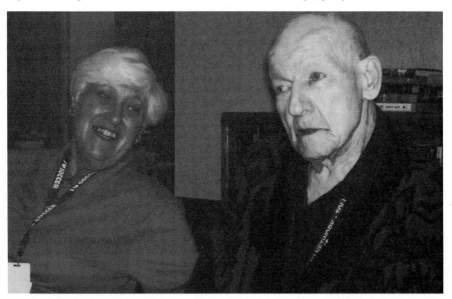

decrease depression, loneliness, and isolation. What is more, through the use of our social work skills to engage the facility as client, we can use both groups and other life-affirming programs to help change the culture of the institution to that of a more humanistic and caring community.

There are many practical considerations that make starting a reminiscence group a great way to begin to shape your own vibrant social work practice in your nursing facility. In this chapter, I will discuss some of the theoretical elements of reminiscence and show how life review applies as a clinical intervention to developmental life-stage issues and how it pleasurably enhances residents' self-images and improves their ability to deal with adversity. I will give a few examples from my own practice of how this theoretical perspective can be translated into clinical interventions. Finally, I will discuss some concrete steps that you can take to develop a reminiscence group in your facility and some further applications of the life-review process.

The nursing home environment is not a given; it is a social invention. The environment by itself does not demand conformity nor ignore individuality. If this happens to be the case in many nursing homes, it is because communities have not expected otherwise; because government regulations, though well-meaning and positive in many ways, have promoted uniformity; and because as professionals we have not imagined, and consequently created, a different reality (Schafer, 1994).

Forming a reminiscence group is an effective way to imagine and create a different reality and bring a measure of psychosocial support to residents. It is also a good place to begin a nursing home practice of program development. Reminiscence work is a particularly appropriate intervention for seniors. Reminiscence touches the core of what makes a person's experiences unique and speaks to the way that such experiences have been integrated into his or her concept of self.

When structured in an organized manner, reminiscence sessions are known as a form of therapy called "life review." Informal life review is said to take place naturally, especially at midlife and late in life as we try to make sense of our existence in the face of an increasing awareness of our own mortality (Gibson, 2004). The beauty of having a structured program that actively engages nursing home residents in reminiscence is that in facilitating a naturally occurring process, we not only assist them to access more fully the developmental benefits of this activity, but also, by strengthening their sense of self, we help them to cope with the losses of health and independence, friends, family, and role identity that occur in an environment that bears little or no resemblance to their former living situation.

Reminiscence work can have an effect on the way elders view themselves and the way that they are viewed by others in the facility. The very act of focusing on who, exactly, these residents are creates a small shift in the way people in the nursing home system relate to each other that may, in time, become an impetus for the transformation of an institutional culture from within. Although the formal authority to mandate the change from a medical model of care to a social one may reside in corporate offices far away, with executives who may or may not consider it important, social workers on the ground level can promote the fundamental concept of interest in and respect for the individuality and life experiences of each nursing home resident.

In addition to all of the above theoretical reasons, one of the concrete reasons why a life-review group is a good way to begin this process is that it is a very enjoyable and emotionally rewarding experience for both the group members and the group leader. Inevitably, the material that seniors choose to remember from the multitude of their life experiences not only is of great personal significance to them but is extremely revealing about the essence of their characters. The process of sharing and listening to such memories is therefore an intensely moving and unpredictable experience that heightens one's feeling of connectedness with others' basic humanity. Such experiences of connectedness as having a former group monopolizer patiently explain to new members that we speak only one at a time, or hearing a resident excitedly tell his family members about how much he looks forward to group meetings, or seeing group members seeking each other out on their own time, or having your group members insist on having group holiday parties and celebrations are not soon forgotten.

A great source of training for social workers interested in reminiscence groups and their applications is the work of Susan Pearlstein, the executive director of Elders Share the Arts (ESTA), an organization founded in 1979 and dedicated to the use of creative expression as a means of promoting healthy aging. The methods that this group has created involve gathering oral histories from participants through specialized guided reminiscence activities and drawing on these memories to create visual, theatrical, musical, and written works that can then be used to validate publicly the participants' lives and achievements, as well as to build intergenerational bonds based on this shared experience. While not purporting to be traditional therapy, the method by which autobiographical material is elicited and the creative act of synthesizing this into a personal narrative is a healing experience in its own right. This organization currently holds experiential workshops in several states and has published several useful how-to books that provide step-by-step instructions for powerful techniques for eliciting reminiscence material, as well as ideas for further developing this material in arts programming with a very high therapeutic value. In particular, an early work published by ESTA about their Living History Theater program (presently out of print) and its successor, *A Stage for Memory* contains excellent structured life-review exercises and interactive group exercises based on theatrical techniques.[1] Presently, ESTA is one of many organizations under the umbrella of the National Center for Creative Aging, a group that Perlstein cofounded whose mission is to identify, link, and promote model arts-related programs for seniors and to serve as a clearinghouse for information about training and resources related to this topic. This group has been engaged in research in association with the National Endowment for the Arts and George Washington University that empirically validates the positive connection between seniors participating in arts programming based on their life experiences and these elders' physical and mental well-being (Cohen, 2006a). These programs tend to promote community among participants and can also be used to facilitate intergenerational relationships between seniors and youth as they engage together in the process of making art that celebrates the lives of the participants.

In addition to being enjoyable and having great clinical value, reminiscence groups are a good place to begin to develop a transformational nursing home social work practice for several practical reasons having to do with patterns of social interaction in the nursing home. For one thing, reminiscence groups are considered to be "traditional" social work and, as such, are understandable and acceptable to the facility. Therefore, a social worker is unlikely to meet with much resistance in starting this type of group, as long as she is careful to explain the clinical benefits of a reminiscence group program to her administrator and interdisciplinary colleagues. At the same time, a savvy social worker can engage other departments in this endeavor by enlisting their support and collaboration in the process of recruiting group participants and working out the details of the group's operation, as well as by sharing information about group members' accomplishments with the staff to enhance their understanding of the residents as individuals and to pique their curiosity about the residents' lives. Being a perpetual cheerleader for new programs and a relentless champion of the residents' identities can result in a great deal of good-natured teasing, as well as perhaps a little bit of annoyance on the part of the staff, but in the end, you are likely to be seen as a committed worker, and after much time the results of your interventions may well earn you the trust and respect of key colleagues, coworkers, and superiors that you need in order to carry out your work. One of the desired results of these efforts is that the entire staff becomes more involved in engaging in informal life-review conversations with residents on their own and in sharing information about who these people really are, resulting in a sea change in terms of facility values and mores. A reminiscence group can be a social worker's entrée into a new role: that of change agent.

Finally, the benefits of a reminiscence group in terms of decreased resident depression and increased socialization can be evaluated by the social worker and presented as a social-service contribution to the facility's quality improvement program. Moreover, the individual results of program participation can and should be documented in the patients' care plans, and such documentation can demonstrate the value of program development to on-site and corporate administrators. Likewise, positive surveys by inspectors from the department of public health in their annual survey process can show that such programs are a very efficient and effective use of social work time, sometimes even more fruitful than traditional casework in reaching residents who may feel threatened by direct clinical interactions.

LIFE REVIEW

While reminiscence and life review are gaining increasing acceptance as having therapeutic value for elders, in particular, many writers define reminiscence and life review in different ways, which makes the literature difficult to understand as a whole. It is possible, however, to adduce some common themes. As one author stresses, memory never replicates an exact event, but is a process of seeking "wholeness or harmony" which causes our minds and imaginations to rework and reinterpret aspects of our pasts that are significant to us into a story that we can accept (Gibson, 2004). A life-review protocol consists of several sessions carried out around questions designed to elicit memories in a structured manner, often chronologically, from early childhood to adulthood and beyond. Thus, each session may cover a particular period in the life cycle. Alternatively, the leader may choose to organize the session around a particular topic—proudest moments, seasons, or holidays, for instance. Typically, a group leader conducts a semi-structured individual or group interview around questions that she has prepared in advance.

A great deal of the literature on the use of life-review groups in nursing homes was written between the late 1960s and the 1990s. Possibly, interest in this subject was a result of the excitement generated by Robert Butler's groundbreaking article, "The Life Review: An Interpretation of Reminiscence in the Aged" (1963). However, life review never became an integral part of social work practice in nursing homes, where it was practiced by social workers on a limited basis, at most, as part of the recreation department's repertoire, conducted as a social activity with therapeutic value rather than as a clinically oriented program ("Remember when they used food-rationing coupons? What did they look like?" "What was the price of gas in 1940? What kind of car did you drive back then?").

What is more, based on my observations and the reports of my senior colleagues, the involvement social workers have had in this endeavor seems to have practically vanished with the advent of subacute care—the practice of nursing homes admitting patients on a short-term basis for rehabilitation under Medicare reimbursement, then discharging them. The current focus of nursing homes (and their social workers) has shifted for financial reasons to the care and management of this population, and as a result, clinicians spend a great part of their day and effort managing their cases and planning safe and appropriate discharges with collateral services such as Visiting Nurse Associations, among others.

However, the benefits of life-review programs more than repay the time required to implement them and help redress the imbalance between short-term subacute care and the long-term care of the frail elderly. Guided reminiscence and structured life review aim to help people to see themselves as rooted in the context of their familial and ethnic heritage and to help them explore and bear witness to each other's triumphant moments, poignant losses, and significant relationships. It enables them to make meaning in their lives. The process of telling one's story addresses the late-life developmental need to work through feelings about past events in order to help resolve what Erik Erikson describes as the crisis of the conflict between "integrity" and "despair and disgust." Erikson's eight stages of psychosocial development each involve the negotiation of age-related tasks and achieving an optimal balance between two possible outcomes. For example, in the first stage (trust versus mistrust, which occurs in infancy), we are dependent on our caregivers and must develop a relationship with them that will consist of a healthy balance of trust and mistrust. The successful resolution of this life crisis results in the individual acquiring the character strength of hopefulness and sets the tone for future relationships. Ultimately, in old age (the eighth and final stage, integrity versus despair), we face the challenge of our mortality and ideally emerge from this life change with a sustaining degree of integrity and only a moderate degree of despair, thereby acquiring the beneficial quality of "wisdom." Erikson further defines wisdom as "involved disenvolvement," an existential sense of self that involves both the individual "I" and mutual relationships with others (Erikson, Erikson, and Kivnick, 1987, pp. 32–53).

When elders tell their stories to another person or a group, it allows them to review their life experiences and construct them into stories that fit and define they way they choose to conceptualize their existence. In the best-case scenario, they come to accept the totality of their experiences, having synthesized them into their own personal epic narrative containing the elements of character and theme development, adventure, pathos, and ultimate triumph over the forces of negativity. In the best-case scenario, this story provides them with a feeling of resolution and completion and even frees them to have hope for the future, however time-limited that future may be.

Even for those of our clients who may have made mistakes in life, as human beings do, we can help them find meaning in life by supporting them in facing their shortcomings and by validating their ability to change the endings of their life stories—to have hope for the future, despite their advanced age. It is human to want to feel that our lives have meant something. It is necessary to our well-being to have hope. We can help them shape their stories with this in mind. Life review can help to heal our wounds and mitigate our sorrows.

If you think about it, the process of life review is what Ebenezer Scrooge undergoes in Charles Dickens's *A Christmas Carol*. Scrooge reviews his life and finds it horribly wanting, but as a result of his dreams of Christmas past, present, and yet to come, he is able understand how he came to lack the capacity for empathy and friendship as a result of his lack of interaction with caring parental figures. He is able to revisit and accept the fact that he had been a miserable person in every sense of the word, someone who has exploited others and behaved as though immune to human emotion. This allows him to come to terms with his regrets and, at the eleventh hour, achieve integrity and avoid despair and disgust. Moreover he is able to use his new insight into the effect of his past behavior to perform good deeds, connect with others in a meaningful way, and, in a sense, revisit and repair some of the earlier developmental tasks that were left unresolved in his life. Seen in Eriksonian terms, these encompass all of the stages from the initial struggle to achieve the trust of others up to and including generativity, the penultimate phase and the fulfillment of a midlife need to contribute to the well-being of the next generation. The result of his process of life review is the resolution of the final developmental conflict that, despite his outwardly indifferent attitude, clearly troubles him and that makes him an unpleasant individual who pushes away anyone who tries to get close to him. Thus, it is a charming surprise and the conceit of the novel that the unlikely Scrooge can accept the sad and difficult fact that he had wasted much of his life, then go on to use this knowledge to inform his actions in a positive way. Dickens's character constructs a meaningful story out of an unhappy existence, a story that enables him to avoid feeling that the forces of life have overwhelmed him, and instead, ending up feeling empowered and able to go on to make a significant difference in the lives of others. Life review can be a redemptive activity.

In our own way, we as social workers hope to achieve a little bit of this grace when we engage nursing home elders in life reviews. As a result of addressing their developmental needs through life review, elders are able to assume the mantle of respect that comes with their traditional role as keepers and teachers of our cultural heritage. As group leaders, we can assist them in stepping into their rightful social position by respectfully receiving their knowledge and letting them know that we appreciate the opportunity to learn from them. Then, as they become aware that their contributions are valued, they may be able more freely to impart the accumulated wisdom of their life experiences with others, including their families and caregivers.

Following are two examples of the way in which telling stories about their lives in a group setting has helped residents place themselves more comfortably in the psychosocial world that they now inhabit.

Albert on "The Love of Your Life"

In this vignette, a small, informal group of World War II and Korean War veterans (all men) discuss their marriages. A couple of the men never married. Albert, a cognitively impaired patient, nevertheless is able to discuss the fact that he remained single all his life and his feelings about this.

Albert: I never got married.
Leader: Did you have an important relationship in your life?
A: I had a girlfriend. Her name was Mary. We met at a dance. I liked her very much. I used to take her to football games.
Leader: Was there a particular reason that you didn't get married?
A: I didn't make enough money. I didn't feel I could provide for her.
Leader: Would you make that decision again if you could go back?
A: Yes, but I wish I had married.
Leader: That is a regret for you. What about being married do you think that you might have missed?
A: The companionship. . . .
Leader: It sounds like you may have been lonely at times.
A: Yes.
Leader: But now you have us.
A: Yes, you are my friends, I like coming here.

Albert was able to mitigate his sadness about this perceived lack in his past with the reassurance that the group that he valued provided him with at least some of the relational connectedness with others that he felt he had missed. Thus, the leader used this opportunity to validate the corrective experience that the patient's positive involvement in the present group provided. In this way, just as Scrooge's transformation did not change his past but enhanced his outlook and sense of well-being, Albert's feeling that he belonged in the group was able to bring him satisfaction that improved his mood and his coping. Albert subsequently discussed his regret with the nursing staff, who assured him that he had women who cared for him in his life at the present time. He continues to come to the group; as his cognition declines, he is less verbal, but he expresses his feeling of belonging with a bright smile that makes his face seem to glow.

Mr. K Finds His Place

Mr. K is a seventy-eight-year-old veteran with Lou Gehrig's disease. He is alert and oriented but has difficulty expressing himself due to the disease. Mr. K is married and has three children. His wife visits regularly, but prior to attending a life-review group, Mr. K attended few activities. He did not socialize with his peers on the unit, and his affect was sad. Mr. K was previously a gregarious man who owned a barbershop as well as a couple of racing dogs. It was his hobby to go to the race-track with his wife to watch them run.

Mr. K agreed readily to attend the group and did not miss a session. As the group got to know him, it became easier for us to understand his slurred speech, and we realized that he had an excellent memory and a great sense of humor. He loved telling jokes and discussing his experiences behind the scenes at the race-track. As a result of his attending the group, he became friendly with his neighbor next door, also a group member. The social worker shared some of his life experiences with the staff, and when it came time for the activities department to take its annual trip to the racetrack, Mr. K and his wife were in attendance. As is the custom, a race was named in honor of the soldiers' home, and the activities director gave the trophy to Mr. K, who was photographed with his wife, holding his prize. It was a proud moment of recognition that Mr. K did not soon forget.

In ways such as these, the process of life review helps elders to account for their lives, celebrate their triumphs and accomplishments, express their regrets in order to resolve their feelings about them, and develop the ability to see their lives as cohesive wholes. This, in turn, enables them to strengthen their sense of personal identity and to give and receive love more fully in their interactions with others.

REMINISCENCE FOR PLEASURE AND SELF-IMAGE ENHANCEMENT

In life-review groups led by social workers, nursing home residents are encouraged to talk about their lives, something they might not often have occasion to do in an environment where their medical needs are paramount and where the focus is on their bodily functions. When one must always focus on one's illness and medical symptoms, there is no opportunity to experience oneself in a pleasurable way. Thus, it is a corrective experience to relive past life events with others there to bear witness and to validate one's past life roles. It can help residents to reestablish their self-concepts. The following is an example of the multidimensional way in which that process can play out. It involves the same group of veterans described above.

The men were discussing their experiences with their first-grade teachers. Frank had described his first-grade classroom (creaky wood floors smelling of a particular disinfectant soap, wooden desks with inkwells where he dipped a girl's braids, black chalkboard). He had described his first-grade teacher (tall, thin, wearing long skirts and bearing a dour countinance with steel-gray upswept hair) when the following interaction occurred.

> *Frank: My first-grade teacher sure was mean. She hit me with a pointer for talking too much.*
>
> *Leader: Why did she hit you?*
>
> *F: For talking too much.*
>
> *Leader: Who were you talking to?*
>
> *F: I was talking to my friend John. We were talking about baseball. All we were doing was talking. These days, kids bring guns and knives to school. What we did was nothing.*
>
> *Leader: So it seems unfair looking back. How did you feel at the time?*
>
> *F: A little scared I guess. (Laughs ruefully.) There was just nothing you could do about it. . . . Yeah, that time my hand swelled up the size of a baseball. We had spaghetti for dinner that night, and I was trying to eat it with my left hand. My dad noticed and asked me why. It's kind of hard to eat spaghetti with your left hand, and it kept falling all over the place. I said I fell on it in the playground. I was afraid he'd go beat up the teacher if he found out. . . .*
>
> *Leader: So in your case, you were protecting the teacher.*
>
> *F: Yeah, I really was afraid he'd beat her up. That's the way he was.*
>
> *Leader: So you felt a lot of responsibility at a young age.*
>
> *F: I guess so, yeah.*
>
> *Leader: What was that like for you?*
>
> *F: It was just the way it was. I didn't think about it.*
>
> *Leader: I'm kind of reminded of the responsibilities that you guys had in the service, in World War II. Some of you have talked about how you were in charge of a lot of men, in positions of real authority at a very young age.*
>
> *F: Yeah, in the navy I had forty men working under me. I was twenty-one. It was kind of awkward supervising men twice my age. But I was their boss; they had to listen to me.*

Leader: You all had to do dangerous things at a very young age.

Bill: We just did it.

Leader: Do you notice any similarities about the stories?

B: It seems like we all did what we had to do.

Leader: You did. It seems to be kind of a theme. You quietly, stoically accepted responsibility even if you were a little scared inside. You had to grow up very fast in a way.

George: I was just eighteen when I joined the army. I couldn't even drink.

F: We couldn't drink, except maybe near beer, and we couldn't vote, but we could fight in a war.

Leader: But you found a way to drink. . . .

F: Yeah, we distilled alcohol from the fuel by straining it through a loaf of bread. We cut off the ends and poured the liquid through it. They put a pink dye in the fuel, so we ended up calling the drinks "Pink Ladies." The captain couldn't understand how come there were so many drunken men on the ship when there was no alcohol. That they knew of, anyway.

Leader: Well that's another theme we talked about. A lot of you drank a lot of alcohol. (General agreement.) Why do you think that was?

G: It was fun.

Larry: It made me feel good

F: I used to drink too much. Now I don't.

Leader: So if I could sum up some of the themes, as a group you pretty much all dealt with some similar issues. About the responsibility, beginning in childhood, protecting your first-grade teacher, or protecting yourselves from physical punishment, and continuing through the war, where you definitely had to grow up suddenly, you just kind of accepted it, there wasn't anyone you could really talk to about it much. And another thing is that a lot of you mentioned that you relied on your buddies and had kind of a "code of silence" not to get each other in trouble. And finally drinking, when you were a little older, a lot of you said that it helped with the stress, at the time. (Pause.) Did anybody else have a similar experience with a teacher?

L (grimly): Yeah, I had the same teacher, a few years later. (Grimaces, shakes his head.) She was something! Mean.

Leader: Did you get in trouble, too?

L: Oh yeah. I was quiet, tried to stay out of trouble. . . .

G: Those days, if your parents found out that you got a beating from the teacher, they'd give you a beating all over again.

Leader: So in your case it seemed that there was no one to turn to?

G: Well, it was like that for everyone. These days, kids know their rights—
they would call DSS. In those days, the teachers could hit kids, and they
did it all the time.
F: We have a lot in common. We've all been through sort of the same things.
We had
nothing, and we made do. We fought for our country. And now people take
things for granted.
Leader: We can take things for granted because you fought for our freedom.
You are heroes.
B: The real heroes didn't come home.
Leader: The real heroes are right here. But we have to stop for now.
F: See you tomorrow! (The group spontaneously claps.)
Leader: Yes, give yourselves a hand. You deserve it!

In this example, the clients were dealing with many issues at once. We began by talking about early experiences with authority figures and touched on how these veterans dealt with authority and responsibility in their adulthood—during the war, as well. The material that was brought up suggested themes for many possible future sessions, including a further exploration of the topic of authority from multiple points of view and the roles they have held with regard to this issue, all topics with the potential for enjoyable discussions.

Encouraging the veterans to view themselves as people who had similar life experiences decreased their sense of isolation. They shared laughter and a sense of connectedness. Validating their accomplishments enhanced their sense of identity and self-esteem. Thus, the session brought them a feeling of joy in the moment.

Feeling fully alive and engaged with others is important, but in addition to being often enjoyable, the benefits of life review can extend beyond the group meetings to the development of connections and friendships with others in the facility outside of these designated times. As these group members got to know each other, they often tended to socialize outside of the group. In doing so, they became more sociable and interactive, visiting with one another on their wards, at functions, and even seeking each other out if they were mobile. As they became more engaged with others, their mood improved, which in turn led to new friendships with peers and staff members and increased positive interactions with their families. In this way, pleasure and image enhancement in reminiscence group therapy can lead to increased coping and decreased depression. The social worker should be mindful of documenting this type of positive result in group members' care plans and progress notes, as evidenced by resident and family reports and staff observation.

PROBLEM SOLVING

Besides being a source of fun, the group can also serve as a resource for dealing with problematic events and as a vehicle for remedial action. To make this possible, the group leader ought strongly to encourage intragroup bonding, so that group members can be a source of support for each other. For instance, when someone in the group is sick or in the hospital, we all sign a card to send to that person. When someone in the facility has died, we use the session as an opportunity to grieve this loss. What follows is an example of the use of reminiscence to address the issue of loss.

The veterans' group was discussing the recent death of a patient at the facility. This death followed a rash of deaths, particularly on one unit that had left residents and staff stunned and overwhelmed. This led to reminiscence about how group members coped with the deaths of friends and neighbors in their lives according to their various religious traditions.

> *Bill (of Polish Catholic background): We never left a body unattended. I remember staying up through the night when an old lady in my neighborhood died. She was just a neighbor, but it was the right thing to do.*
> *Leader: Where did you sit?*
> *B: In the parlor.*
> *Leader: What did the room look like?*
> *B: A regular room. Chairs, couch, wallpaper, flowered curtains.*
> *Leader: What did it smell like?*
> *B: A musty smell.*
> *Leader: What sounds did you hear?*
> *B: It was very quiet, just the clock ticking.*
> *Leader: How did you feel?*
> *B: She wasn't someone I knew very well. I felt sad that she had nobody, but good that I was doing the right thing.*
> *Leader: Yes, that was very kind of you. Have other people had similar experiences when someone died, or were your traditions different?*
> *Dominick (Italian Catholic): When someone died, the body was waked at home. I remember when my grandmother died, the body was in the house for three days. It was hard, as a kid, being around so much death and crying. There wasn't a break from it like there is now, when people go to funeral homes. . . .*
> *George (Irish Catholic): The Irish drank. That is, the men drank downstairs, and the women cried upstairs.*
> *Leader: How did that make you feel?*

> *G: When I was a kid, I felt scared, seeing all the women crying, and when I was older, I drank with the men.*
> *Leader: Did that make you feel better?*
> *G: At the time it did.*
> *Leader: But in the long run, did drinking solve the problem of sadness and loss? (G and others admitted that it had not, that there had been times when they drank excessively, and that now they had quit drinking.) Can you think of other ways that we could mourn Chris's death and celebrate his life?*

Mark suggested that we might name something after him and put up a plaque. Bob suggested sending a card signed by all to Chris's family. We sat for a moment in silence for Chris, which ended with by Mark's solemn proclamation that we would never forget him. We talked about the things that we would not forget, good and bad—his kindness and generosity, giving away his money and possessions to his family and friends, his bravery during the invasion of Normandy, his braggadocio and constant interrupting of others. The group ended by clapping. "Chris, this is for you," someone said, "wherever you are."

Staff members told me that while the group members did report some relief after this session, a feeling of unresolved sadness lingered. Some of the nurses reported that this took the form of increased acting out on the part of the residents, particularly on one of the units where a lot of men had recently died. This prompted me, the unit social worker, to work with the administration, the hospice service that was contracted with the facility, and my colleagues on the interdisciplinary team to develop a systematic protocol for dealing with death and bereavement at the soldiers' home. I will describe this further in chapter 8. Suffice it to say for the purpose of this chapter that my intense engagement with the group led to an awareness of their feelings that galvanized me to become more involved in their lives and to work with others to seek alternative solutions to their problems. In this way, as has been the case time and time again, the vitality of an effective program also had a catalytic effect on the group members, on the staff witnessing the changes wrought by the group, as well as on me as the group facilitator. This caused me to exert my influence further to change what formerly had been a fairly sterile environment into a more humanistic setting where the lives and deaths of the community were recognized and honored.

Life review provides an opportunity for frail institutionalized individuals to feel a sense of mastery over their lives by tackling the developmental challenges they face and also to improve their quality of life through meaningful social engagement with others, important achievements that are related to positive health outcomes (Cohen, 2001). Additionally, the synergy that results from engaging residents and staff members in developing and implementing a life-review group has a significant effect on changing the focus and values of the institution as a whole from the medical management of sick and old people to a vibrant therapeutic community where elders hold a respected role.

CONDUCTING A LIFE-REVIEW GROUP

In general, the basic recipe for a life-review program, as for any program, is to have a structure—a flexible structure. This means having a concrete plan, but not insisting on sticking to it if it is unsuccessful at sparking the group's sustained interest. A good way to start is to plan and execute a time-limited group. This gives the facilitator a chance to experience the process and generates a feeling of success when the goal is reached. Small successes are the building blocks of a successful practice, one with several ongoing programs and other innovative interventions. About six weeks is a reasonable period to debut a life-review group.

Where to find the time for such a program can seem like an insurmountable obstacle. No one would argue that social work time is limited. There are many meetings and duties that are fixed and mandatory parts of the social worker's schedule. There are crises and emergencies that absolutely must be attended to, ranging from acute psychiatric situations to upset family members. Your beeper will go off in the middle of a meeting, and you will be called to deal with a family member suddenly faced with the decision of whether or not to have their loved one who can no longer eat be placed on a feeding tube. This will necessitate imposing yet again on a co-leader, perhaps a volunteer who you don't want to overburden for fear she will quit, or perhaps it will require making hurried arrangements to end the meeting and bring the residents back to their rooms, enlisting a passing staff member with whom you have a good relationship to help, if you are lucky. In addition to the inevitable interruptions, there is a significant amount of documentation that cannot be ignored. All this is a given. However, if a social worker checks her schedule carefully, there may be a day and a time that is less busy than others—an hour and a half or so with no planned meetings—when she could consider holding a reminiscence group.

A word of caution: the social worker should try to make this an immutable portion of her schedule, as unalterable as care planning and other administrative meetings. She should carve out this time and let staff know that she is unavailable

for anything else except a dire emergency. She should let the switchboard opera-
tor know not to page her unless it is absolutely necessary. She should also enlist
the support of the administrator and director of nursing in this endeavor and, if
possible, convince a staff member, possibly the activities director or assistant, a
nurse, the administrator, or the occupational therapist, to help plan and execute
the program. Contracting with the facility to work together on this program for
six weeks helps ensure that others in the facility will have ownership in the
process and will increase the chances that life review and other creative ways that
the social worker might devise for addressing clinical goals will be incorporated
into the daily routines of facility life.

REMINISCENCE GROUP THERAPY: CONTENT AND PROCESS

In practicing life review with nursing home residents, I have used as my starting point the *Life Review Training Manual* (originally published by the National
Center for Creative Aging and now out of print, superceded by *A Stage for Memory;* see note 1). The processes by which life-review material is elicited in ESTA's
programs (Living History Theater and others) belong in the toolkit of every group
practitioner, especially those working with an older population. Moreover, suitably extended, these exercises serve as the basis for programs in drama and the
visual arts which also have significant clinical value.

Structured life review helps seniors understand themes in their life roles by
exploring these in an organized manner—for example, chronologically (for example, beginning with early childhood memories, then moving on to memories of
the ages five to ten, ten to fifteen, fifteen to twenty, and so on). When discussing
the group participants' memories at each particular age, it is important to have
an particular topic, for example, "Games that I played at age five to ten," "Where
these feet have gone, age eleven to fifteen," "A major life transition when my life
changed direction, age sixteen to twenty." One also can focus on the same age
span and explore a variety of topics, such as family relationships, school and work
roles, or hobbies. Props can be used to trigger forgotten memories. So can photographs, music of the participants' generation, food, or things to smell, such as
essential oil with a pine smell, cinnamon, Ivory Soap, ice, snow, metal keys, or
motor oil. Colored objects or colored paper, photographs featuring a particular
color, or things to touch (a baby blanket, grass, silk, sandpaper) can do the same.
In discussing people's memories with them, it is important to help them "set the
scene" by recalling all of the visual, auditory, olfactory, gustatory, and tactile
details they can about the place where the particular event that they are remembering occurred. Such questions as "What did the ballroom look like?" "What

sounds did you hear?" "What were you wearing?" and "What smells did you smell?" would be appropriate for the social worker to ask when discussing someone's memory about attending their first formal dance, for example. In addition, it is important to reach for relationships associated with the event. Such questions as "Who was there (or not there)?" "What did they look like?" "What were they wearing?" "What were they doing?" and "How did you feel about that person?" are key to understanding the nature of the bond between the storyteller and important figures in his or her life. Similarly, people's perception of their roles at various stages of their lives can be clarified by devoting several reminiscence sessions to this topic. One way to do this would be to ask what their roles in the family (such as "peacemaker," "leader," "nurturer," "clown," etc.) were at different ages (five, ten, fifteen, twenty, etc.) and ask them to give an example of a situation where they performed this role, complete with sensory detail and details about other significant figures involved in the situation they describe. This exercise is useful in helping participants identify themes in their personal relationships throughout their lives that might persist into the present time. This may lead individuals to decide if they like these roles or wish to change them, as did Scrooge did following his life review.

A exercise in this manual designed to evoke fundamental sense memories is one of its signature creations, entitled simply "Going Home." This guided reminiscence is significant because of the importance of the concept of home to our sense of selfhood. Home signifies belonging, safety, family, and comfort. The concept of home is particularly poignant to institutionalized elders, who, due to physical frailty, have lost their most recent home and are disconnected from a sense of belonging that was shaped by their experiences in their childhood home and further developed in the homes that they created for themselves as adults. Engaging in a group reminiscence session, sharing one's experiences of home, and identifying with and being validated by others can help to restore symbolically what has been lost. According to Nora Rubenstein, "Sometimes there is no way back home, no way to belong except in imagination. But there are also times when reminiscence and fantasy morph and merge, when past and future interpenetrate, when imagination and longing may enrich us, protect us, save us, and that interpenetration may be a creative act" (2005, p. 112). Thus, remembering one's home(s) can be a way to reconnect with the past.

The process of returning home in imagination, as described in the *Life Review Training Manual* involves many of the elements of structured life review we have discussed, including the use of sensory detail, and a focus on life roles. This powerful exercise is conducted as follows:

Exercise

Take a deep breath and close your eyes. Imagine you are five (ten, fifteen, or another age) and you are going home. Imagine the walk home. What do you see/smell/hear? As you approach the house, notice its shape and color. What is it made of? How many windows does it have? Are there stairs leading up to the house? What color is the door, and what is it made of? What does the doorknob look like and how does it feel in your hand? As you open the door, what do you see? What do you see (smell, hear) as you walk through the house? Go into your favorite room and pick up your favorite object. What does it feel like? Now, when you are ready, take a deep breath and open your eyes. Who is ready to tell us about their house?

When using this technique, the social worker is in effect identifying, developing, and validating thematic content related to Erikson's life stages. When clients bring up material pertaining to significant relationships in their lives, significant events, or seemingly mundane interactions that in fact describe and define the meaning of these relationships to the individual, the social worker can begin by exploring these events and their attendant sense memories with the individual group member and then extend the discussion to include the related experiences of other members. In this way, participants can begin to process the meaning of these events in the larger context of their lives, gaining additional perspective on their own experiences by comparing them with those of others in a supportive environment.

In order to ensure that the environment is indeed a safe one, the social worker must be prepared to deal with the aftermath of the session and with unresolved business, such as grief. Moreover, the social worker should also be aware of the dynamics of the group, observing both verbal interactions and such nonverbal communications as body language and facial expressions. She can then make appropriate interventions as indicated. These include encouraging reticent, passive, or cognitively impaired members who tend to be overlooked to express themselves, if only briefly, if that is what they can tolerate, so that they can feel included. Additionally, setting limits on those who would dominate the conversation and prevent others from contributing is sometimes necessary. The social worker can do this by summarizing the statement of the long-winded member, validating its content, and then directing the focus of the conversation to someone else. The social worker should also be sensitive to the need to defuse potential conflicts and to prevent escalation of negative interactions by acknowledging feelings and enforcing a group norm of respect toward others. Above all, it is crucial to maintain an atmosphere of safety, support, and mutual regard.

Setting Goals and Objectives for a Life-Review Group

When starting a life-review group or any type of therapeutic group, it is important to have clear goals and objectives related to the particular needs of the client population. For instance, the social worker may wish to address the needs of residents in the nursing home who are alert and oriented, yet isolated and depressed. While nursing homes are admitting more and more individuals with advanced dementia, those who are relatively intact cognitively often have socialization needs that are not necessarily met by large-group activities such as bingo and restaurant outings, where they often do not have the opportunity to connect with their peers on a meaningful level. Frequently, these individuals do not want to socialize with the others because they do not want to be considered "old" and/or "sick" like "them," and they note that they find "them" too depressing. In fact, it is a frightening thing to be faced with the indignities of aging and dementia, and in response, some people understandably try to defend themselves against their fears by avoiding "them" like the plague, as if the symptoms of confusion and infirmity were, indeed, contagious.

For the more alert people, a negative dynamic occurs. Perhaps some elders initially did not socialize because they were distressed about being in a nursing home to begin with, especially with others who appear to be more impaired than they (accurately) felt themselves to be. This, in turn, engenders a situation in which the new residents isolate themselves to the point where they become depressed, irritable, unpleasant, and consequently disliked by the staff. These people can be fine candidates for a life-review group, where their past roles as fully functioning individuals will be validated, which can often boost their self-esteem, increase their coping, and decrease depression—incidentally, all good goals that can be noted in their care plans. Often, the effect of such groups is to increase the participants' sociability to the point where they eventually feel comfortable interacting with other group members, new residents, and even their more impaired peers.

Deciding on the Structure of the Group

The group's structure ought to be decided in advance—for instance, whether the proposed group will be an open one, in which any clients can drop in at any time, or a closed one, in which new members will not be admitted after one or two sessions to ensure continuity as members get to know each other and share their experiences. Since one is never sure if the group will be successful or require adjustments, it is a good idea to stipulate in advance whether it will be held for a limited time or limited number of sessions. After this, the facilitator can terminate the group as scheduled or decide with the group (and with the permission of the administration) to continue, and if so, whether to admit new members or even to open the group to all on a more informal drop-in basis. It may turn out that having such a group could be a good way of helping new long-term residents truly adjust to their environment and make new friends. The leader should be cautious about admitting short-term patients to the group; the dynamics in this situation could be difficult, particularly because these individuals may be appropriately focusing on leaving the facility and returning home, something that is not an option for the long-term residents.

Selection of Group Members

Selection of members for a group should be a careful process. Generally, eight to twelve participants is a good number for life-review groups because it is large enough to have a variety of different viewpoints, yet small enough so that everybody gets a chance to speak. To facilitate communication, group members' particular needs, such as hearing, need to be taken into account. The social worker can make adjustments such as using a microphone if the residents' hearing aids are not sufficient to allow them to participate fully in the group.

The social worker can use her own judgment in selecting participants, but also solicit referrals from other staff members. The process of asking for referrals from the nursing department, for example, has the benefit, from a strategic point of view, of engaging key players in the nursing home system in the process and of encouraging their investment in the success of the group.

The leader must take into consideration certain traits or characteristics of potential group members that would make them either a good or a poor fit for the particular combination of individuals in question. Including different individuals with a range of cognitive functioning is workable in a reminiscence group, but individuals who are disruptive or who wander would be poor candidates for this setting. If residents with mild to moderate dementia are included in the mix (and with the current trend toward a nursing home population where this diagnosis predominates, this is necessary and appropriate), the social worker should take care to ensure that their cognition is such that they would not feel overwhelmed by the demands of participation in such a group. She should also include a number of alert, oriented, and extroverted individuals to help keep the conversation moving along.

In considering group dynamics, the social worker should be careful about accepting a group member who has a known tendency to dominate social situations, especially if he or she might be resistant to redirection. This is not to say that such individuals might not be able to be managed in the group, but the social worker should use her judgment about whether she and any possible co-leaders could reasonably do so.

Contracting with Prospective Group Members

To ensure that prospective members obtain the maximum benefit from the experience of a time-limited life-review group, it is useful to sit down with them beforehand and explain the goals, purpose, and format of the group in language that the resident can understand. One can describe how the group will be talking about "old times" and "some of the important things you have done in your life, such as your job, and your family, beginning in childhood, all the way up until now." The social worker can say that she thinks the client will enjoy this chance to make new friends and find out what he or she has in common with others. She can relate that many people find that participating in a reminiscence group helps them to feel better physically and mentally. The more enthusiastic you are about the program, the greater the chances are that your excitement will be contagious.

In addition to talking about the goals of the group, the leader(s) should be clear with each potential participant about the expectations of the group. These include the fact that their attendance is expected for the specific number of sessions that the group will meet. Moreover, confidentiality should be briefly touched on in positive terms, such as, "This group will be confidential. What is said in the group will stay in the room, except if you give me permission to share information, and except for certain special conditions related to safety." Finally, something should be said about the group having ground rules that will help to make it a caring and safe environment for all.

If after some version of this discussion the resident is willing to participate in the group, this is a verbal contract. The agreement can be further formalized with the resident by signing a brief written contract. This may help to emphasize the fact that the resident will be participating in a special program, distinct from their other activities, and to concretize the resident's commitment to the undertaking.

The Setting

The room where the meetings are held ideally should be removed from the commotion of the nursing units, but close enough that transportation is not overly difficult. The task of bringing the residents to the group can be an onerous one in that it is most often the case that no one is available to assist the social worker. Certified nurses' aides are often unable to assist because as they are busy with the residents' personal care. The challenge of transportation also applies to programs held by the activities department. Therefore, the social worker can take her cues from the activities director as to the logistics of this process. It is advisable to develop a good working relationship with the activities director to solve problems related to this issue. In this matter, as in all other aspects of social work, relationships are the foundation of our practice.

The seating arrangement is something that should always be considered. In general, a circular arrangement is helpful in promoting an atmosphere of inclusiveness. If you plan on serving coffee and refreshments, arranging the tables into a square usually works well.

A Word on Refreshments

Refreshments tend to increase attendance at any meeting. Getting coffee and snacks requires making arrangements with the kitchen. The activities director, who works closely with the dietary department in planning food-related events, can again be helpful in negotiating with the food service director. It is important to know which patients are diabetic and which may have swallowing difficulties so that appropriate food and thickened beverages can be provided. At the soldiers' home, I learned to have a can of thickener available for residents who require this. Since sweets are not recommended for diabetics, we often served fruit cocktail, which is healthier and which almost everyone can eat, because it is compatible with a diet for individuals with mild to moderate swallowing concerns.

Meeting Times and Length

Usually no longer than an hour is appropriate for a reminiscence session because attention spans may be limited due to cognitive losses or other factors. In general, it is better for the clients to have a positive group experience that is a little too short than one that is longer than they can tolerate. In the first case, they will be eager to come back for more, whereas in the latter situation, they could be overwhelmed and unwilling to return. In terms of meeting times, it is crucial to stick to a regular time and date as much as possible, even though this is quite challenging, so that it can be counted on by the residents and the staff. This helps to ensure that group members feel that their time is valued and that the group is a predictable and safe environment. Emergencies do arise that may necessitate cancelling a session, but it is essential for the social worker to make continuity of her program a priority in her schedule and to be respectfully assertive with other staff members and the administration in doing so.

Rules, Group Norms, and Values

To ensure that the life-review group is a predictable and safe environment, some basic rules need to be established from the start, while, on a less formal level, the development of group norms and values needs to be fostered as the group progresses. Confidentiality, as I previously noted, is an important baseline rule and needs to be articulated as such. This includes letting the group know that the facilitator(s) will not share the specifics of sensitive information with the other staff members without first asking permission from the individual involved, as well as encouraging the group to let "what is said in the room stay in the room" and discouraging gossip about group members outside of the group.

Respect for all participants is a rule that needs to be strictly enforced. This means making it clear that there should be no interrupting when someone else is talking and letting the group know that it is necessary to share the floor so that everyone who wants to do so can have a chance to participate. Those who do not wish to speak should not be required to do so. Moreover, to ensure that everyone is treated with dignity, group members must be told to refrain from making negative comments about others. They can be taught to communicate their feelings about what is said through the use of "I" statements, letting other members know how they feel about what is said, rather than expressing their responses in judgmental terms.

Closely related to group rules are group norms and values. These are created over time. As the members of the group get to know each other, they develop certain ways of relating to each other that define the culture of the group. Positive group attributes should be encouraged by the leader(s). These include valuing both commonalities that group members share and the differences between participants. The leader(s) can then reinforce these values throughout the sessions by encouraging members to try to distinguish common themes in the stories they share in a particular session and to notice differences in other peoples' stories, experiences, and their emotional responses to these. The leader(s) can support group members as they empathize with each other about happy as well as sad life events by gently prompting them to share accounts of similar situations, to express how they felt about this, and to discuss how, as a result, they are aware of how the other person felt and may still feel. Leader(s) should provide validation when other members spontaneously express empathy and make statements that indicate that they are beginning to consider the group as a caring community.

Opening and Closing the Sessions

Generally, it is helpful to have a small ritual for opening the group sessions. This can be elaborate or simple, based on theatrical techniques such as purposeful breathing or on a standard greeting that the group leader might devise. For example, "Welcome to the Tuesday Morning Reminiscence Group. Last week, we discussed our memories of Thanksgiving dinner, and many of you mentioned how wonderful it felt to sit at the table with your extended family and share special dishes prepared for the occasion. Today, I thought we might further discuss our favorite relatives, and tell a story about them. . . ." This simple opening provides reassuring continuity and has the added benefit of demonstrating to the group members that their contributions have been remembered and will form the basis for further discussion, providing them with some measure of control in an environment where their control is at a minimum and institutional routines prevail.

Again, to close the meeting, a simple ritual such as holding hands, repeating a selected phrase ("Until we meet again" or "Thank you for coming and being with us today") can be effective. For some reason, one of my groups always ends with the group members clapping, and at that point I (or a co-leader) adds: "Give yourself a hand." This is now our ritualized way of acknowledging each other and thanking each other for our contributions. It may sound corny, perhaps, but it brings a smile to our faces.

Documentation

Keep a notebook in which you can record attendance and keep notes on the content of the sessions. This is helpful when writing quarterly notes and may prove useful later in evaluating the program. It can also serve as a resource should you ever wish to use the material in a scholarly way. Also make notes in group members' care plans of their participation in the group and document their responses to the group in their quarterly progress notes. You may find that writing these notes gets easier and less time consuming because you get to know the group members quite well and don't need to search the chart to find out about their psychosocial concerns.

Terminating the Group

As was mentioned earlier, when the six weeks (or other number of contracted sessions) are over, the social worker may terminate the group as planned or decide to continue for a specific number of sessions or time period. In either case, the last of the initially contracted sessions is a time to review with the group what the experience was like, how they felt about it (good and bad), what they learned, how they benefited (or did not), and how they feel about the time being over. Particularly if the decision is made not to continue at this time, group members should have an opportunity to discuss feelings of loss that this might entail, and the social worker should validate these feelings and relate them to other losses that the group members might have experienced. She should also point out that the members of the group can continue to enjoy the friendships that they have made, and she should encourage them to attend activity programs where they can continue to socialize with others. The last session is a time to serve special refreshments and to celebrate the accomplishment that the elders have made by completing the life-review program. At the end of the last session, certificates of completion can be presented to the participants as a commemorative souvenir.

Even if the social worker and the group decide to continue to have further sessions, it should be acknowledged that the program in its original format is ending and that this represents a change and possibly a loss. However, in this case, the social worker can emphasize to the group how further sessions can present an opportunity to meet and get to know new residents. It is amazing how institutionalized elders can live on the same unit, eat at the same table, and even sit together in front of the television or nursing station for years without ever talking.

Evaluating the Group

In order to evaluate the success of the group in addressing depression, the social worker can take pre-group and post-group measures of participants using the Folstein Mini-Mental Status Exam, a brief fifteen-point questionnaire with yes/no responses that can be administered verbally or in writing to individual participants. Additionally, the social worker may wish to compare indications of depression on the routinely administered Minimum Data Set assessment that is completed by the facility as a requirement of the department of public health. Furthermore, the comments of participants and the observations of the staff and family members can all be considered in evaluating the program. Keep a record of such comments in a notebook, along with your notes on the group, so that they will be handy when needed.

In evaluating the effect of the program on the residents' physical health, the Minimum Data Set assessment tool can again be used. In this case, look at the sections devoted to functioning in the areas of the activities of daily living (bathing, dressing, etc.) and nutritional status. Additionally, the data about the residents' number of medications and hospitalizations before and after program participation can be compared. This is an ideal project for a quality improvement report, something that many social service directors are expected to submit on a quarterly basis. Finally, documenting a successful program helps to legitimize the practice of creative program development as an effective, efficient means to affect positively the patients' health and functioning.

A Word on Working with Co-leaders

When working together with another facilitator, if you should be so fortunate, maintain excellent communication with your colleague and discuss, even if briefly, how each meeting went and any plans for the next meeting. I have found this to be particularly important when the relationship between co-leaders is the least bit problematic. It helps the co-leaders to stay focused on the goals of the group and gives them a structure, which helps them to work together more harmoniously.

OTHER USES OF REMINISCENCE

The potential value of life-review programs in social work is great and remains to be developed. In the context of the nursing home environment, it can be as helpful in meeting the institutional needs of the social worker and of the institution itself as I have found it to be in meeting the psychosocial needs of long-term residents.

A nursing home social worker can use residents' biographical material to help staff members understand and value these people as individuals. One way to do this is to interview a resident or their family, with the resident's and family's written permission, of course. Their biography can be published in the facility newsletter, for example, with photographs from the subject's past. This can give a resident who does not normally receive much recognition a significant boost in self-esteem; staff members, residents, and families tend to read the facility newsletter and often come to compliment someone who is featured in the publication. Having their loved one featured in the paper is also validating to families and helps them to overcome some of the normal and expected guilt that they might experience about placing a loved one in a nursing home. Having their relative's life publicly honored signals to his or her family and other families that the facility is a caring one. It can also help the facility maintain a positive relationship with a family who may at times be seen as critical or demanding toward staff members and/or the administration. Finally, an awareness of residents' backgrounds sensitizes staff members to the reality that the residents they are caring for are truly complete human beings who have led full lives, something that is unfortunately easy to forget in a medical environment. Thus, the personhood of their patient becomes real to them, and the patient can no longer be easily dismissed as the cranky old person in bed 203. In my job at the soldiers' home, I made it a practice to contribute a monthly article about a resident to the newsletter, accompanied, if possible, by pictures from the resident's military career or other aspect of his past, such as holding a great-grandchild on his lap, displaying a memento of a cherished hobby, or looking dignified in his current setting. More recently, I have involved nursing assistants in writing these columns, which I take to be a sign that a cultural change has begun.

LIFE-REVIEW GROUPS AS SYSTEMIC INTERVENTIONS

Whether the social worker decides to stop or not after completing a time-limited number of sessions, holding a reminiscence group is a tremendous accomplishment, and she should be proud of it. Doing so is a systemic as well as clinical intervention. To hold a group, the social worker must consider the nursing home itself, with its various departments, its many layers of administration, and its medical-model culture, to be a secondary client. In working with the system as client, the social worker must, as always, form alliances that will be the basis for her work. Moreover, in intervening on a systemic level, she can promote the existence of a holistic therapeutic community where perhaps none previously existed. Indirectly, this larger intervention will help to create a nursing home culture that values relationships and that helps to restore the individual and group identities of frail institutionalized elders who have lost their homes, their possessions, their positions in society, their health, their mobility, their vision, and their former social networks. This function of social work may not be not spelled out in one's own facility's social work job description, but it is implied in our professional code of ethics:

> Social workers recognize the central importance of human relationships. Social workers understand that relationships between and among people are an important vehicle for change. Social workers engage people as partners in the helping process. Social workers seek to strengthen relationships among people in a purposeful effort to promote, restore, maintain and enhance the well-being of individuals, social groups, organizations and communities. (National Association of Social Workers, 1999)

A social worker is an agent of change.

Note

1. *A Stage for Memory: A Guide to the Living History Theater Program of Elders Share the Arts* can be ordered at www.creativeaging.org/publications.htm by downloading an order form and mailing it to: Elders Share the Arts, 138 S. Oxford Street, Brooklyn, N.Y. 11217, phone (718) 398-3870.

Chapter 4

The Art of Social Work

ALTHOUGH MANY SOCIAL WORKERS HAVE AN APPRECIATION OF OR INTER-
est in the arts as spectators or participants, only a few venture to use these skills
in their practice. However, as I have discussed in the previous chapter, the growing success of programs for seniors that make use of the arts, such as those
endorsed by the National Center for Creative Aging (NCCA), give credence to the
psychological benefits of integrating one's life story into a form of creative expression, as well as the value of using the arts as a means of developing community
among isolated elders. Anecdotally, I have found my own intuitive efforts to
explore ways to incorporate my previous training in the visual arts to be useful in
enlarging the range and scope of my interventions, as well as enriching the depth
and quality of my engagement with my residents, the connections I have been
able to encourage them to make with their own pasts, and the bonds that they
have been able to forge with others in the process of art-making. What follows is
an account of my own career-long efforts to incorporate the arts into my work as
a nursing home social worker.

This account may even be of interest to those social workers who feel that
they have little or no affinity for the arts. Some of the simple programs I have
developed may give you the confidence to try these ideas on your own or consider
engaging a professional artist to work on with you. Alternatively, you might find
applications for your own special skills and interests. For example, someone very
skilled in the use of computers might think of innovative ways to connect with the
residents through this technology, as well as explore ways in which the residents
could use computers to connect with their families and the larger community.
The point is that the art of social work is the inventive use of oneself as a therapeutic intervention to meet the multidimensional needs of one's clients.

In the 1980s (before it became too dangerous), I sometimes took my exercise
in the form of a run around the quite beautiful local cemetery. At the time, which
was before I entered a graduate school of social work, I was searching for a way to
gain experience in the medical field. One day, on completing a circuit of my usual

route, I noticed a "Help Wanted" sign in the window of the small brick building across the street. Curious, I walked into the first nursing home I had ever entered. I remember my first impression was that the place seemed dark and dim, but oddly cozy, with its ruffled curtains, strong smell of disinfectant, and bare, but clean, institutional corridors which reminded me of my old elementary school. It was a family-owned nursing home, something that very rarely exists anymore. The job on offer was that of an assistant in the recreation department. The activities director, Mark, a pleasant and ebullient young man, was wheeling a cart bearing the remains of what looked to be a giant coffeecake. Staff members and some of the ambulatory residents approached him, and he jovially handed out pieces of the rich pastry. Everyone seemed to draw cheer from his company. Frail-looking seniors appeared to brighten in his presence. The staff, who had been bustling about purposefully, suddenly became friendly, bantering and joking with Mark. Intuitively, I sensed that everyone was hungry for more than cake. They were looking for someone or something to make this odd place of care a real home. Mark seemed to provide that missing ingredient.

Mark's office was full of half-finished crafts and handmade chocolates. There were signs of meaningful life here. I found it irresistible. On a whim, I asked for the job and was hired on the spot. Thus began my lifelong love affair with nursing homes, a love affair that is not without its ambivalences, sadness, frustrations, and, yes, joys.

I found that it was, in fact, easy to make the residents smile. All you had to do was smile yourself, and they smiled back. I was young, and they liked that. They were like grandparents to me. As a child, I liked my own grandparents, but they had lived far away, and I saw them infrequently. Many of the residents in the nursing home loved to talk. They painted word pictures, and their stories brought the details of ordinary existence to life. I learned about how the iceman delivered the ice in a horse-drawn carriage to homes where families placed a little card in the window, signifying whether they needed a five-pound, ten-pound, or fifteen-pound block. They placed the ice in a box to keep their food cold. It lasted about three days. A black gas stove kept the kitchen warm in the winter. They used coal to heat the house, and when it was in short supply, during the Depression, they gathered it on the railroad tracks.

In the activities department, we were in charge of giving some value to life. The nurses checked vital signs, passed out medicines, and called doctors. I don't recall the social worker even being around much, unfortunately, except that he did attend meetings and interact with the administration. The medical staff minded the body. We in activities minded the spirit.

We brought the patients to church on Sundays, and I stayed while Hank, one of the residents, pounded out the hymns on the piano and the rest sang enthusiastically. This was a meaningful tradition for them, and I sensed the comfort they took in it, even if they were squabbling as soon as they were out the door. Other times, we played bingo and brought out apple and German chocolate cakes from the walk-in freezer for endless "coffee hours." We baked and cooked, the Italian women calling out instructions and admonitions about how to break the eggs, mix the batter, cut the vegetables.

While these things brought some collective comfort, there seemed to be a need for personal expression. We needed a way to connect these people to the persons they truly were, both individually and as a group. Because I was trained in art, it seemed like a natural thing to try with them. I gathered a few of them together. I brought in shells I had collected at the beach, and we drew these, learning to observe and interpret what we saw with lines and shadow. Then we did self-portraits. George's was strong and bold. Lilly's was delicate and observant. They made portraits of each other. Struggling with the question of whether to "put in the wrinkles," they settled more often than not on a solution that mixed kindness with candor and that preserved both their self-esteem and their friendships. I displayed the results on the bulletin board. While participating in my "classes," the residents realized themselves individually and bonded as a group. Some were quite talented and went on to make more artwork—still lifes in watercolors. Their creativity gave me a sense of an authenticity that was often lacking in this artificial environment, something that they could express at church and occasionally at coffee hour or bingo, but rarely on the units, where concern over bodily functions ruled the day. To bring forth something novel and creative is to be alive—still.

Arts and traditional crafts are powerful tools to reach the elderly so that the elderly can reach themselves and experience a sense of relatedness. For many residents, working directly with their hands and using traditional materials seemed to connect them with memories of their own life experiences. We experimented with quilting. Sewing came into the conversation. As it turned out, this was a rich topic of discussion for the women. Many of them had sewn and even worked in the garment industry. Some of them now began sewing and crocheting on their own, making gifts for their families and the staff. I still treasure a hand-sewn clown that a resident gave me more than twenty ago. I imagine that the other staff members and families treasured their gifts, as well.

For the men, woodcrafts reminded them of some of the things they did around the house, building and fixing things. Although sanding and staining simple objects was often a challenge physically, the process of making something was richly satisfying, as were the conversations we had while we worked. All of this culminated in a wonderful craft fair that Mark organized, open to the community, with the residents' finished products proudly displayed and made much of, with additions from Mark and me making up possibly the bulk of the inventory. Residents helped to man the tables. The production was complete with raffles, homemade pies, and ice cream. This yearly event, which was much anticipated and looked forward to by all, coincided with the Christmas season and seemed to be the time when residents, staff members, and family members came together most visibly as a community.

In 1995, several years after graduating from social work school, I was working as a director of social service in a medium-sized nursing home owned by a large corporation. A sense of community was definitely lacking there. It was a difficult place to work, politically. There was a high turnover of staff members, as well as administrators. We were not operating at capacity, and we all felt the pressure from corporate to "fill the beds." Meeting followed meeting. I remember suggesting to the administrator that we market to the Russian community, which was prominent in the area. He did so with some success. For my reward, it seemed, I was told that my job was on the line. But then, so was everyone's. Poor surveys from the department of public health meant that fingers were pointed and blame flew. One major issue in the mix was the execution of safe and effective discharges, something that required close coordination between the rehabilitation and nursing departments to develop a check-off form to ensure that no detail was overlooked. It was truly a learning experience—a trial by fire. In that fire, I forged my skills.

In between trying to plan systematic discharges and survive in a somewhat dysfunctional system, I thought back to the warmth and sense of togetherness I had felt in my first nursing home as an activity worker. I wondered if I could somehow make a difference by making changes to this corporate environment, an environment that seemed so impersonal and distasteful. I reflected about art and how it had brightened the walls with an uplifting sense of human potential in the displays that I set up in my first nursing home. I decided that here, too, the walls could use some art. With the most recently arrived administrator's permission, I organized an exhibit of local artists.

I called and wrote to local art associations soliciting artists to show their work at the nursing home. The theme: local landscapes. About seven artists responded. We set up a show. We sent invitations to staff members and residents' families and placed ads in the community and metropolitan papers. We invited the residents, as well. A sumptuous buffet served as a draw. The artists came and talked about their work. The response in the facility was very positive. The residents were interested and loved the paintings. We even got a musical dividend; a volunteer offered to play the piano, and the event became even more engaging. The residents served as judges and picked their favorite painting, which received a blue ribbon. (I got the prize, but then, I am pretty sure that they knew it was my work.) Afterward, the paintings were for sale and hung in the dining room for several months. They transformed a functional room into a vibrant space.

A few years later, in another nursing home, I found myself frustrated with what seemed like an excessive amount of emphasis on documentation, as opposed to getting to know who our residents were. The director of nursing, a lovely but inflexible woman, had a firm belief in the "right way" of doing things that seemed to me to have more to do with "paper compliance" with department of public health regulations than anything else. Along with others in administrative positions, she would brook no deviations. In addition, there was a lot of factionalism. Staff members actively and openly disliked one another personally. These two dysfunctions were perhaps related. In a rigid system where mistakes were not tolerated and blame was freely distributed, friction among members of the staff seemed inevitable. Needless to say, the system was not good for the residents. They were bearing not just their own problems but the issues of the self-wounding nursing home.

In this hypercritical atmosphere, I began to learn how to make a valuable social service contribution to the interdisciplinary team. Focusing on my responsibility to know my clients, I employed a method developed by David Danforth to organize information, biographical index cards about each one of the residents (David Danforth, personal communication, July 1998). I worked hard to memorize their ages, diagnoses (with particular emphasis on psychiatric labels), and medications (again, paying special attention to the psychotropic). I came prepared for care-plan meetings with pertinent facts about the residents' social histories, such as ethnic background, marital status, number of siblings, level of education, military service, occupation, number of children, and hobbies and interests. In sharing this information with the team, I gradually began to distinguish myself on the team as someone with information about the residents' backgrounds and personal characteristics and eventually was able to make contributions to team meetings based on this knowledge that assisted the team in developing personalized solutions to identified problems. Eventually, this enabled me to stop worrying about the question of my competence—the question that was, for this nursing home, the order of the day.

In the process of working to define and demonstrate my social work role, not only did I gain extensive knowledge about my residents, but I learned to connect with them as individuals who had held a variety of life roles. Learning their stories gave me a format to engage them in rich conversations about their past. The index cards helped me to put the focus back on social work, as opposed to letting the system define me or my job.

But there was another, serendipitous dividend: I was brought back to art and the inestimable value of creativity for the elderly. Getting back to basics in my social work practice led me to notice that a fair percentage of my index cards indicated that several members of this population had had some involvement in the visual arts. It occurred to me that there might be a way of validating their past artistic identities and making others aware of their individuality by honoring the rich artistic community that actually existed, unrecognized, in the nursing home population.

I decide to have an art show, this time not the works of outside exhibitors but of the residents' own past work. I asked families to bring in some pieces of their loved ones' artwork from their collections. The families were excited that their relatives' work was being valued and appreciated. The paintings themselves were amazing. Some were intimate portraits of children and nature done in a sensitive, realistic style. Others were fresh and individualistic, such as the landscapes in vivid colors done by a woman who began taking art classes at a mature age at her local senior center. I still remember one painting where the pale, almost florescent green of budding leaves evoked the first weeks of spring. How different the painters of these diverse and personal works seemed from the uniformly fragile and medically compromised seniors with their walkers and wheelchairs. Aside from honoring these people for their artistic achievement and allowing others to see the world as they saw it, the object was to present the elderly as unique individuals whose visions of life and the world were worthy of continuing respect, not merely old people whose lives were nearly over.

The title of the show was: "The Way I Saw It." Once again, I obtained administrative approval at the facility for a display of the residents' works in a prominent public location, the local library. Picking a few choice canvases, I made an appointment at the library and solicited their approval for this project. The community relations representative was enthusiastic, and the event was a great success that was written up in the local paper.

Despite the triumph of this one project, and no matter how well and truly I had engaged the residents and the larger community, in the end the facility continued to malfunction as usual. My crusade to humanize the hospital-like environment had failed. Moreover, I continued to feel alienated from my peers and their concerns. The problem, as I came to understand it, was that I had not first built a base of support at the facility. I had followed my own agenda, and as well suited as it was to enhancing the well-being of my clients, it had not been in synch with the culture and mores of the facility. I needed to learn to develop alliances with the other workers if I wanted to use art as a vehicle for positive change with any degree of success.

My first attempt to involve interdisciplinary staff in an art-related intervention did not actually involve an art program but took place on an individual level
to address the needs of one particular patient. In this case, many team members
collaborated on an intervention when an eighty-five-year-old woman named Suzy
became tearful and depressed after she had a stroke and could no longer crochet.
Here, the entire staff was mobilized around a shared concern about a psychosocial issue, for this woman's depression about her loss of creative functioning was
affecting her appetite, sleep, and motivation to participate in the activities of daily
living. It was clear that if her mood did not soon improve, her health would be
adversely affected. For once, I was able to share ownership in the process of using
art as a therapeutic intervention with the team. It was truly a group effort.

First, we obtained a selection of simple crafts from the activities department.
Then, with the help of an occupational therapist, we found that Suzy had sufficient range of motion and fine motor control to make intricate designs of colored
beads and that when these were warmed (by the rehabilitation staff with a hot iron
under protective paper), they formed unique and interesting pieces. Often, during
the day, the nurses on her unit would set up Suzy's art materials on a tray table
in front of her. While she was working, the tearfulness stopped, and Suzy's mood
improved when she received much praise for her creations. Everybody was
pleased with this resolution of the problem.

This intervention was much more of a success than my previous efforts
because I had been mindful of the need to include the institution as client, as well
as the resident, by deliberately emphasizing the strengths and resources the other
departments. This time, our joint success provided a foundation for future artistic endeavors. In this spirit of working creatively in collaboration with others, I
approached the activities director, MaryAnn, about developing an art program.
Together, we appealed to the administrator for permission to apply to the Massachusetts Cultural Council to participate in their (now unfortunately defunct)
ElderArts Program.[1] When she agreed, we wrote the grant for an artist to come to
our facility weekly for twelve sessions and develop a program based on our
requirements. Laura, who was the artist that the ElderArts Program provided,
MaryAnn, and I decided to call this program Cycles of Life.

The aim of Cycles of Life was to engage the residents in life review through
the arts. We believed that the use of art was important because it would heighten
the experience of reminiscence through the use of the senses. The residents
would incorporate touch, sight, and even sound into the act of creating artworks
based on their life experiences. Moreover, they would have a finished product by
which to remember the experience. To validate the residents' sense of accom-

plishment further, we proposed that the sessions culminate with a celebration that would recognize their work—and ultimately, their lives.

Since a requirement of the grant was that the progress of the project be documented, we decided to ask the local cable station to televise the art classes. There was no cost to us, and Chelsea Cable generously showed us how to edit our tape. As a result of being on television, the residents received even more recognition from the local community. This publicity also added an element of excitement for the staff and, importantly, was congruent with the facility's goals because it served as a marketing tool. Thus, the program was of interest to staff members and of value to the administration.

Highlights of the meetings with Laura included the residents creating dioramas on the theme of the ocean. They used shells, sand, found objects, and cut paper to reconstruct their memories of the sea, sometimes while listening to music that evoked a particular era in their lives. The artist photographed their work, and the results were visually stunning—a beautiful product for them to display and keep. Another important piece involved the creation of collages celebrating important achievements for the residents. One woman depicted herself in a nurse's uniform, reflecting her sense of accomplishment at having gone back to school at age fifty and earned a nursing degree—after having raised nine children. Another woman made a collage about her wedding. All of the residents were pleased with what they had accomplished. The tape made by the television station caught their emotions as they shared their work with the group and described what it meant to them. At the end, as planned, we held a reception for our artists and their teacher. It was a joyous event, attended by families, residents and staff members, and the artists basked in the recognition they received.

Another project that I collaborated on with the activities director was to apply for a grant from the Massachusetts Department of Public Health for funding that actually comes from penalties collected by them as fines for failing to comply with the regulations. Together, we developed an intergenerational project, the goal of which was to have the residents, particularly the men, mentor local children in a Salvation Army after-school program, children who often grew up in homes where fathers were absent. On alternate months, we visited the children and the children came to us. The residents helped them with crafts projects, such as building birdhouses and making Christmas decorations. We also had the nursing home staff bring in cans of food for the Salvation Army to distribute and sponsored holiday parties for the residents and children. In the course of our meetings, the children became very comfortable with the seniors, who greatly enjoyed and looked forward to their visits.

Some programs in the arts can be started without the benefit of a grant. In the soldiers' home, we started a photography club. This idea came to me when a new resident remarked, during his initial psychosocial assessment, that he loved to take pictures. This resident was not pleased to be admitted to a nursing home and expressed his displeasure with his family and caregivers with a variety of provocative behaviors. My activities director, Dan, and I gave him a disposable camera, and he shot a roll of film, including pictures of his family, his dog, the outside of the facility, and scenes from a field trip to the shore. He was very pleased when I printed these pictures for him. After that, we kept him supplied with cameras, and his pride in his work gradually led him to become less irritable with those around him and to take an active part in the many trips and other activities that Dan provided.

With the activities director's support and financial assistance (because the recreation department has a budget and social services does not), I supplied cameras to other residents, who also took pictures. Some of the residents required assistance due to dementia, but they enjoyed the process of taking pictures and seeing the results of their work. All expressed an interest in participating in a club, so we scheduled an initial meeting. The small number of residents with which we began grew into a group of ten to twelve photographers that met

Figure 3. Photography group picks out pictures for a show.

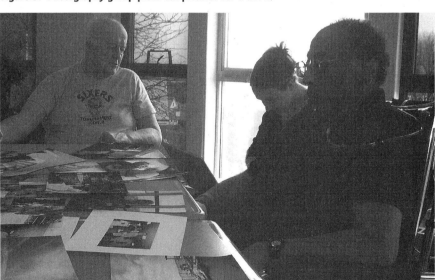

monthly. We were joined by some of the veterans from the independent dormitory who happened to be avid shutterbugs. Katie, a graduate student in photography and the granddaughter of one of the participants, volunteered to teach the group. Her enthusiasm and gentle manner made learning new skills unthreatening and fun for all. The residents were enthusiastic when we presented a show in the activity room that combined Katie's sensitive portraits with their own photographs of each other, their family members, the staff, and their pets.

Eventually, we applied for and received a grant through the local cultural council to cover the expenses of used digital cameras in lieu of the disposable kind, as well as a small stipend for our instructor as a token of appreciation. Currently, we are preparing for another show that we hope to open up to the larger community, in which the veterans would not only share images representing their current lives but also images of their earlier lives and military service. The intent of this project is, of course, to validate the identities of those who so often are seen in the role of patient rather than individuals (in this case, warriors) who have had a myriad of roles and responsibilities.

In any case, the monthly meetings of the photo club have proven to be an efficient and effective way of extending social services to a number of residents simultaneously. My relationship to these residents tended to be more authentic and positive than when I was simply responding to problems, administering paperwork, or providing check-ins to residents I did not know well. In terms of the benefits to the facility, social work art programs can be counted by the activities department as evidence of resident involvement. These programs are also useful to the administration in terms of marketing the unique qualities of the facility to prospective customers. Not least, they will impress inspectors from the department of public health.

As you can see, creative interdisciplinary collaboration can be used on an individual level to address the concerns of a particular resident, as well as in therapeutic art programs. Moreover, these examples demonstrate that art programs need not be delegated solely to the activities department. Instead, social workers can use the arts in their own work while engaging others in an interdisciplinary endeavor that quite directly addresses the holistic needs of the residents.

I have found that projects tend to grow in an organic process that seems to take on a life of its own, and therefore I can offer no real recipe for creating programs that are not specific to each particular environment. However, it is important to prepare the objectives and logistics of the initial project carefully and to plan for possible future developments. Once the project is started, it is best to try not to control too rigidly the direction the project will take, to be open to new ideas, and generally to go with the flow when it comes to the process of the group meetings. A necessary condition for success is the social worker's consistency and persistence in making the meetings happen.

It is a good idea to keep notes on attendance and the content of the sessions. This documentation helps validate the importance of the program and is useful when analyzing the objective benefits of the program. Furthermore, participation in the program should ideally be documented in residents' care plans in terms of how it helps them work toward their psychosocial well-being and mood- and behavior-related goals.

Many of my colleagues tell me that they do not have time to do extra projects, let alone something much fun as an art program. To this, I respond that, in my experience, doing this enjoyable work can actually save time. Like life review, it can save time trying to document the care provided to clients whose ways of relating to the world, outside of their daily routine as a patient, are unknown to you. Not only do you get to know the participants in an art program really well, but you may have the added benefit of being able to do informal rounds, chat with other residents, touch base with staff members, and become privy to the latest crises de jour on the units, all in the process of gathering residents for a group. In some cases, art programs can even save time working on behavior plans and documenting problems because participation in psychosocially meaningful programs positively affects people's mood and behavior, eliminating the need to write extensive care plans.

Besides economizing on time, using the arts can save energy in that working together creatively with others in turn provides social workers with a more positive workplace experience that replenishes the spirit. Not all of us are or even want to be artists. However, I hope that the story of my journey to integrate creative expression into my practice will inspire and assist you in finding ways to incorporate the universal language of the arts into your work, in order to help nursing home residents to rediscover, or perhaps discover for the first time, their own unique voices and in using your own talents and interests creatively to forge connections and develop community where none previously existed.

Note
1. Although the ElderArts Program no longer exists, a related program called Healing Arts is being run by the Massachusetts Cultural Council in partnership with health care facilities. I strongly encourage social workers who are so inclined to partner with other staff members, particularly activities directors, to bring the community's local artistic resources to their sites.

Chapter 5

Specialized Resident Programs

IN PREVIOUS CHAPTERS, WE DISCUSSED PROGRAMS THAT WERE IMPLE-
mented to meet the psychosocial needs of nursing home residents through reminiscence and through the arts. In this chapter we will explore several other types
of resident programs. All of these were designed to validate and enhance residents'
sense of selfhood, as well as to promote general recognition of their individuality.
A by-product of these programs has been to strengthen the development of a
sense of community in the nursing home.

Generally, an institutional system is not designed to value individuality
greatly. As Philip B. Stafford (2003) states, "When you enter the nursing home as
a patient, you experience a loss of self, of personhood. Your walking becomes
'ambulation.' Your food becomes your 'diet.' Your eccentricities become your
'behaviors.' Your life becomes your 'record'" (p. 1). Although nursing home policy
dictates that attempts be made to accommodate individuals' preferences, such as
honoring their bedtime and rising schedules, in practice, altering the facility
timetable for each person is not a priority compared with maintaining a high standard of medical care. Yet even if supreme efforts were made to adhere to aspects
of their previous schedule as reported when they were admitted, how could each
residents' idiosyncrasies truly be known if we as caregivers are not actively
engaged in communicating with the residents, learning about their stories and
the experiences that have shaped their lives? We like to say that the nursing facility is the residents' "home." How can it feel like a home when all of the emphasis
is on the patients' medical problems and we, the caregivers, find ourselves inadvertently referring to people as "Mr. W, you know, the blind man on 4 East" or
(worse) " Mr. G, the trach tube on 5 West"? We need a more holistic approach.

Resident-centered undertakings are one way that social workers can effectively modify nursing home culture from a medical model to a more humanistic
one. Programs can help us to put into practice the values of concern and caring
for our clients as fully sentient human beings, rather than as clinical diagnoses,
and provide a way to involve others in the nursing home system in more authen-
tically human interactions with the residents. At the same time, the elders'

involvement in meaningful activities has been shown to improve their own perceptions of life satisfaction (Calderon, 2001).

In addition to life review and arts-related programs, some other types of programs that can be developed to meet the requirements of specific resident populations include (but are not limited to) programs for Alzheimer's patients, support groups for patients with specific medical conditions, programs for resident self-advocacy, and eclectic groups that meet more than one purpose.

In this chapter we will look at some examples of these types of groups. These include: a multisensory group for residents on a dementia unit; two medically related social work support groups—a stroke support group and a low-vision support group; a residents' council; and a "current events" group that actually promotes reminiscence, cognitive stimulation, and socialization as well as awareness of local, national, and world events.

In order to give the reader a sense of process, we will review in some detail the way events unfolded in the formation of these programs. The process is organic, incorporating roadblocks and barriers into structural elements and taking advantage of "happy accidents," much as a watercolor painter would permit an unintended mark to remain in her painting, the "mistake" being much more interesting than anything originally intended.

A MULTISENSORY GROUP FOR RESIDENTS ON A DEMENTIA UNIT

With a colleague, Donna, the director of the Occupational Therapy Department at my facility, I developed a strategy to provide cognitive stimulation and fellowship to some of our patients, male military veterans on an Alzheimer's/dementia unit. The occupational therapy perspective was key to the success of this group because it focused on the adaptation of the physical environment to meet the needs of this special group of clients. Due to her training, Donna was keenly aware of the cognitive and perceptual limitations of the group's participants. These limitations necessitated breaking tasks down into manageable steps and maintaining a calm environment free from overstimulation, as well as providing materials in bright, contrasting colors appropriate to the residents' visual requirements. Within these parameters, we envisioned this program as a multisensory initiative whose goal was to evoke positive memories for those who had lost the intellectual capacity to process complex thoughts or ideas and to encourage these individuals to interact with each other.

The process by which this program took shape illustrates the necessity of being flexible and deviating from one's original plan in order to reach desired goals. In this case, we initially intended this to be an outdoor horticulture program. We were aware from these residents' histories that some of them had been avid gardeners, while others had maintained a garden at some period in their lives. This led us to believe that they would still be interested in this activity and that this extremely tactile, sensory activity would enable these people to access some memories of happy moments in their lives. Moreover, horticultural therapy has been shown to be particularly meaningful to dementia patients by invoking "procedural and emotional memory," helping them to remember familiar routines that were an important part of their lives (Gigliotti et al., 2004). However, when we began to take steps to put our plans into action, the logistics of getting the residents, many of whom were in wheelchairs, outdoors to the only available gardening location proved to be insurmountable, at least for that year's growing season. Therefore, we decided to put aside our original idea of an outdoor garden until such time as an accessible plot of land could be made available for this purpose. Instead, we made arrangements for several window-box gardens.

Donna and I elected to start with herbs, because of their pungent and evocative fragrances, in order to maximize the potential benefits of aromatherapy. Although Alzheimer's patients are said to experience a decrease in their sense of smell compared with their "normal" age cohorts and are said to be unable to detect certain odors—specifically strawberry, smoke, soap, menthol, clove, pineapple, natural gas, lilac, lemon, and leather—positive sensory stimulation of all kinds has been found to enhance their quality of life and to enhance cognition (Devanand et al., 2000; "Loss of smell," 2004; Brock, 1998).

Since the attention spans of our clientele were limited, we chose to complete only one garden box during each weekly session. For the first meeting, we covered some tables with newspaper and brought out our planting containers, bags of dirt, and seedlings. We crushed the leaves of the herbs between our fingers and allowed everyone to smell the scents, which they enjoyed. "Rosemary goes straight to the back of your throat and lingers there. It's a good smell," one patient noted. We discussed the various dishes that contain this herb, and this led to a conversation about the cooking that the men and their mothers and wives had done, as well as much talk about the vegetables that they had grown on their farms or in their backyards and how this bounty was canned and preserved for the winter and the excess shared with their neighbors.

With our help, the patients took an active part in pouring the dirt, planting the seedlings, and watering the plants. Various family members who were visiting their loved ones on the unit took an interest in the proceedings and volunteered additional recollections about their relatives' gardening accomplishments, which unexpectedly served to enrich the atmosphere of fellowship and community.

Along these lines, another heuristic accident happened during an early session of this group. We had just finished planting red geraniums when a guitar player engaged by the activities director wandered into the solarium where we were gathered and started playing. Taking advantage of the moment to enhance the multisensory focus that was our goal, we asked the musician to play some planting-related songs, and he obliged with "Inch by Inch, Row by Row" by David Mallett, "Old MacDonald," and other related tunes. Thus, the ability to capitalize on unplanned events turned what could have been an awkward interruption into a very special afternoon, one that ended with one patient waltzing in the arms of his granddaughter while others conversed with their relatives about long-ago gardens and some sat peacefully in silent contemplation of the bright flowers in the middle of the table.

When you think about it, many of the best practices in any endeavor involve this attitude of flexible resourcefulness. I believe that the "habilitation" approach articulated by Alzheimer's expert Joanne Koenig Coste is as much about having such an attitude as it is a practice or method. Habilitation involves "validating the patient's underlying emotions, maintaining dignity, creating moments for success, and using all remaining skills" (Coste, 2003, p. 204). Doing so successfully requires what Twyla Tharp (2003) calls "the creative habit." By this, she means being open to using one's own creative resources in a disciplined way in one's practice. In the case of the multisensory group, the purpose of the project was to help Alzheimer's patients, if only for a limited period of time, experience happiness and feel fully human. What better luck could we have had than to have family members present and music to help make this happen?

As our weekly meetings with the dementia unit patients progressed, my co-leader and I sought to continue to make the time we spent with them fun and relevant to their interests. In order to engage their senses, we brought fruits and vegetables to smell, touch, and taste and sampled foods that related to our weekly topics. We also used other props. In addition to the sensory, we strove to stimulate their cognition and socialization. We found that the population we served loved history and facts in general, so we downloaded from the Internet information related to the plants that we were growing and talked with the residents about what we had learned. This accomplished several purposes, as it turned out. Even when they were not able to follow all of the details, which we presented in a simple format and in an enthusiastic, yet low-key manner, the residents were interested in hearing or recalling bits of information, as evidenced by their verbalizations of surprise and comments of agreement or even of elaboration on subjects about which they were previously expert. Thus, not only was the activity a pleasurable one, but it helped to stimulate focus and concentration. Moreover, it addressed the universal need to preserve one's dignity and selfhood, in this case, a dignity and self-possession befitting their status as veterans and men who had once functioned capably in the world.

Collaboration with a colleague from another discipline helped to enhance the therapeutic benefits of the program, as well as to ensure that the initiative was accepted as an integral aspect of the care provided by the facility. Our interactions with the members of the group were not only enriching to them, but gave us as staff members a more grounded understanding of their personalities and cognitive functioning than I could have obtained from simply doing rounds on the unit. Moreover, it helped us develop trusting relationships with these sometimes difficult-to-reach residents. Finally, doing this work enabled us to earn their families' trust as caregivers who know their loved ones and participate in personalized projects with them. In short, a seemingly simple program with the patients on a dementia unit provided a truly systemic intervention.

MEDICALLY RELATED SOCIAL WORK SUPPORT GROUPS

Social work groups related to coping with illness can provide a normalizing context for the anger and grief that result from the psychic insult and injury associated with the loss of functional abilities related to a medical condition. Moreover, such groups provide a support network for their members. The meetings can be a resource in providing education to residents about their condition, thus helping to demystify their diagnosis. Finally, incorporating elements of life review into these support groups can be beneficial because focused self-reflection in supportive group settings has been shown to help elders to decrease their experience of negative emotions, such as sadness and loneliness (Zauszniewski et al., 2004).

The first medical social work group that I initiated was a stroke support group. In the facility where I was then employed, there was a large rehabilitation unit where many patients came to receive therapy following an illness or injury with the goal of returning to their former living situations. Some of these elderly individuals were unable to reach their goal of living independently and therefore needed to stay permanently in the nursing home. A number of these individuals were stroke survivors.

I felt helpless in the face of the raw pain that these people so obviously experienced. As a consequence of their cerebrovascular accidents, many of these patients were emotionally labile, moved at turns from tearfulness to agitation by the frustrations caused by their loss of control over their bodily functions, their difficulties in communicating, and the numerous major life changes that their conditions entailed. Their clear psychosocial needs for a sense of competence and control over their environment, for a restoration of their ravaged sense of body and self, and for a way to renegotiate their roles in their relationships with their loved ones all led to my desire to form a support group to assist them in coping with their situations. I hoped to be able to provide a measure of solace, as well as an avenue for them to pursue self-advocacy and to gain back a sense of efficacy in their lives.

In planning the group, I thought about how it would be difficult for stroke survivors who had to remain at the facility to witness the very different struggles of those who would be able to return to the community following short-term rehabilitation, so I elected to focus on residents with this condition who required long-term care, including both new residents and others who had resided at the facility for some time. Gathering six residents together, I encouraged them to share some of their hopes and goals for the group. Many of these goals seemed unrealistic to me. More than one wheelchair-bound resident insisted that they would like to "walk again" or "go home," despite the prognoses given to them by their doctors and therapists. I did not want to give them false expectations, but I also did not wish to take away the hope that they had. I decided to engage representatives from the American Stroke Association and other resource providers to educate the patients (and me) about the realities of their condition.[1]

From these speakers, we learned that, contrary to the Medicare regulations that mandate that treatment stop when a "plateau" is reached with no visible functional gains over a short period of time, we learned that it is important to find ways for survivors never to stop striving for improvement. Encouraged by this advice, we queried the rehabilitation department for exercises that the group members could perform on their own. Since it was recommended that one group member lose weight in order to increase his mobility, we developed a plan for him to increase his daily exercise and decrease his caloric intake. With the support of the group, he was able to make some positive changes in his lifestyle that both improved his mood and had a modest positive result in his physical functioning.

Along the same lines as encouraging the residents to persevere in their efforts to heal themselves, despite gloomy predictions, I worked with the nursing home to maximize their independence in any way possible. Thus, when the facility dietician started a breakfast club in which residents who were able to do so could go to the dining room during certain hours on certain days of the week and order and enjoy a leisurely morning meal, I encouraged group members to take advantage of this opportunity. I also assisted those who were interested in applying for wheelchair van transportation services provided by the state to plan individual outings with their families.

Over the months, from these residents and following their agenda, I learned the power of hope. As time went on, the residents, motivated by some of their positive accomplishments, began to develop new, more realistic goals for themselves, such as improving their mobility in a wheelchair or standing unassisted, as opposed to the unrealistic goal of regaining all of their pre-stroke capabilities.

In addition to validating the positive things that the group members could do to improve their situations, it was also necessary to address their sadness about the many losses that they had endured. We talked about the frustration of not being able to go home, the frustrations of living in a controlled environment, and how much some of them missed their families. Several patients were quite angry that their spouses and loved ones were no longer able to care for them, and it was helpful for them to express their feelings and to be validated by others with similar experiences. The residents shared ideas for setting limits with overprotective spouses in terms of such issues as making their own medical decisions, enjoying positive marital and family visits, and spending time with their grandchildren. Again, I found the use of reminiscence to be of therapeutic value in helping the residents to validate their life accomplishments. It helped them identify their strengths and the ways in which they had dealt with adversity and had negotiated interpersonal conflicts in the past, allowing them to draw on such strengths and skills as perseverance, faith, and humor and to avoid unproductive coping mechanisms in dealing with their current dilemmas.

Not being sure how long the group would require to accomplish its tasks, I did not set an initial time frame for the number of sessions for the group. After five or six months of weekly meetings, we came to a point where the members were emotionally stable and no longer needed intensive intervention, as evidenced by improved mood and coping and decreased interest in weekly meetings. Since the patients did benefit from the community provided by being with others who had much in common with them, as well as from the friendships that they had developed, when an opportunity for an expanded art program became available, the activities director and I encouraged the members of this group to participate. Thus, most of them stayed together, and the art group became almost an extension of their stroke support group. They also remained friendly on an individual basis.

Theoretically, a group such as the stroke support group could be reinstated should the need arise (although, since I have left that facility, I do not necessarily expect that this would happen). In any case, this example demonstrates the importance of the social worker being in tune with the fluctuating needs of her caseload and using creative program development to address them effectively. In terms of efficiency, the group format involved a relatively small expenditure in time on the part of the social worker, compared with the return that resulted—a documentable amount of decreased resident depression and increased participation in the facility's activities. As well, the group format provided participants with a sense of camaraderie and community that could not be obtained from individual psychotherapeutic visits from the social worker or from the facility's psychiatric service.

A LOW-VISION SUPPORT GROUP

Another example of a medically related social work group is the low-vision support group that I developed at the soldiers' home. Again, it was a population-based need that led me to develop this group. One particular veteran at the facility had a degenerative ocular condition and was experiencing a fairly rapid decline in his ability to see. Mr. G expressed feelings of hopelessness and helplessness at this turn of events. He stated that he felt life would not be worth living if he "went totally blind." I contacted the State Commission for the Blind to see if they were aware of any local low-vision support groups that Mr. G might be able to attend. Because there were none, the commission social worker suggested that I start my own. With her encouragement, I decided to do so. The group, gathered from my caseload, consisted of Mr. G; Mr. D, an amputee with advances diabetes; Ms. R, a woman who had suffered a stroke and had degenerating vision which affected her ability to read and do crafts; Mr. Z, who suddenly found himself legally blind after complications from an unrelated surgery; and several others.

Armed with a list of local resources for the blind that she had supplied to me, I contacted one such organization and was fortunate to be provided with a list of suggested protocols for forming a low-vision support group, including some advice on potential group speakers from various organizations. These protocols are helpful to have as plans or roadmaps in forming your own group, although you may choose at any point to deviate from their format in favor of one more suited to your group's particular needs. The Internet is a fine way to search for resources in your state.[2] You are likely to find that once you make a few initial contacts in your field of interest, you may be referred to other resource people because local professionals in helping communities tend to work together and are familiar with each other's work.

As in the multisensory group for Alzheimer's patients, it was helpful to have a co-leader for several reasons. First, when dealing with a medical illness, it is nice to work with someone who has more knowledge or experience about that condition. Moreover, having a co-leader helps to provide you with moral support, and this helps to sustain the program's momentum. Finally, involving a coworker from the facility is a great way to begin to engage the nursing home in the project immediately at hand and is a step toward the social work objective of developing a community connected by caring for the residents—that is, of treating the facility as a client.

In this case, I took advantage of the fact that I have a visually challenged colleague, our facility priest, Father Healy. I realize that not every institution has such a convenient resource available, but I include this information in the spirit of encouraging others to use their ingenuity in locating possible co-leaders and using their social work skills to develop working relationships that will enable them to collaborate on such projects. In my case, understanding that unlimited monthly attendance is a large commitment to ask of someone, I sought to nurture our collegial relationship by inviting Father Healy to attend the first meeting to determine his level of interest and participation in the group. As it turned out, he graciously agreed to be a facilitator, and he later reported to me that he found the group helpful both as a resource for himself personally and in his mission to be of service to others. He turned out to be a fine and useful co-leader who could relate to the group members on the basis of shared challenges and serve as a role model for them in terms of coping.

At the first meeting, we focused on commonalities that the group shared. Because all were veterans, we included a discussion of their military service. In other nursing homes, one might wish to open with a recognition of other shared characteristics, such as perhaps the residents coming from the same general community of local towns or even the fact that they are all in the same facility. That being addressed, we moved on to talk about their vision loss, when it started, and how it has affected their lives. As the facilitator, I encouraged them to share their individual experiences while also pointing out commonalities and differences in their accounts and those of guest speakers. The veterans' shared the experiences of being in a foxhole at night without the benefit of light or sight, the crushing blow of having your drivers license revoked due to the inability to drive safely, the annoyance of having people greet you and expect to be recognized on the basis of voice recognition alone. One guest speaker, a lieutenant in the fire department, explained how he had taught his men to identify each part of the fire truck by touch alone. And the daughter of a former U.S. Marine described to the residents how, blind from the age of twenty, she raised a family, held a job, and was active in her church, a bracing example for residents who were discouraged over their own failing eyesight in their later years.

As the culture of the group developed, so did the members' coping skills. We all learned to value the comfort of members sharing similar experiences, their ability to learn from how others had coped, and the richness of spirit that the appreciation of others' differences brings to our lives. I urged them to listen attentively and to empathize with one another's feelings about the course of their life events, especially those related to decreased ability to see. The group learned the value of humor for coping when Father Healy admitted that he had once inadvertently blessed a large oxygen tank, leaning forward toward the bed of a sick patient.

Aware of my own limitations in knowledge about various visual conditions, I made it a point to bring in speakers frequently to educate us on the medical conditions that affected the group's participants and on the resources available to them. These speakers included the facility ophthalmologist, who talked about the various kinds of vision loss and the purpose of the various medical instruments in her office; a representative from the Blinded Veterans Association, who discussed veterans' financial benefits relating to the loss of vision; and an outreach coordinator from the state commission for the blind, who, among other things, provided us with a list of state benefits for the legally blind. In addition, a facility dietician spoke to the group about the importance of a healthy diet for maintaining one's residual vision as well as one's overall physical well-being. This resulted in individual requests for such healthy foods as fresh fruit, which were addressed by the dietary department. Finally, a representative from a local school for the blind discussed such assistive recreational devices as books on tape, audio-described movies, as well as possible outings for low-vision residents such as specially guided tours for the blind at the local fine arts museum.

All of this information helped to demystify the condition of blindness for the residents and stimulated them to discuss their situations logically and realistically. Doing so allowed them to view their diagnoses more positively in terms of what they could do, as well as the things they could not. As the participants shared specific medical difficulties related to their vision, they were encouraged by the group facilitator, visiting professionals, and their peers to follow up with their nurses and doctors with the assistance of the social worker and to take advantage of the clinical services available, thus helping them regain a sense of control over their bodies.

A theme that we discussed at the beginning and the end of each of the sessions added structure to the group format: What were some of the challenges they had faced during the previous month, and what were some of the successes they had achieved? At the end of the sessions, we encouraged the group members to reflect on these issues in order to review their progress at the next meeting. This ritual provided a bridge between sessions that helped to sustain the group participants over the coming month.

The benefits of the low-vision support group have been many. Blind or partially blind residents no longer felt alone in their condition and had a renewed sense of hope due to their awareness of resources and services that can help to improve their lives. The group also served as vehicle for socialization. Friendships were formed in this forum, and some residents used the group as a launching pad to go on to attend outings and other recreational activities. A few residents who otherwise attended very few recreational programs came to this meeting, which suggests that it had become an important part of their support network. In addition, as a result of these meetings, the nursing home staff had an increased awareness of residents with visual difficulties, and this helped them to be more in tune with the residents' specific needs. Finally, resources from the outside brought in by the social worker were being integrated into the facility. Various clinics were now more frequently used as referral sources by the nurses for their residents, and the staff developer engaged representatives from local government agencies for the blind as instructors for employee training. The low-vision group became an ongoing feature of life in the nursing home because it continued to meet the needs of the facility.

RESIDENTS' COUNCILS

Monthly residents' councils are mandated in nursing homes. Although many social workers believe that, in theory, the primary role of a social worker in the residents' council should be that of facilitator, in practice, the extent of social worker participation in this forum varies. Some councils are designated as the sole responsibility of the activities director. Since advocating for the residents is a significant social work responsibility, I recommend that the social worker take an active role in participating in this formal vehicle for resident participation in social work policy and procedure. One way to initiate this is to offer to present one or two of the residents' federal and state rights for discussion at each meeting, simplifying the language from legalese to layman's terms that can be understood by all. An example of these rights is the right to refuse treatment. Residents can be coached to ask to speak to a social worker, charge nurse, or nursing supervisor if they feel that their right to decline to take their medication is not respected. They should also know how to contact their regional nursing home ombudsman, if they wish to do so, as well as their local department of public health. In short, by addressing the residents' council, the social worker can promote patient assertiveness in planning their medical treatment with their doctors and the interdisciplinary care-plan team. Although some administrators may be skeptical about advising residents of their rights, it is ultimately in the facility's interest to do so, because the department of public health expects the residents to know this information, and this may be looked into during annual inspections, when the department traditionally calls a closed meeting of the residents' council and solicits the residents' concerns.

If the social worker has the opportunity to have increased input into the proceedings, it may be helpful, depending on the level of cognitive abilities of the population and the receptivity of the administration, to organize the council for increased efficacy. This may include the nomination of a president or co-leaders to help represent the residents' concerns to the administration. It might also involve the social worker helping the residents work together to address any issues that they might have. An example might be preparing the residents to invite the director of housekeeping into a meeting to discuss a prepared list of their most urgent laundry-related problems, having a cordial, issue-focused meeting where solutions are generated, monitoring the result of these solutions, and extending recognition to the laundry department for their responsiveness. Having their voices heard by the management and working together with the home to improve their quality of life is empowering to the residents and promotes positive communication and increased facility responsiveness to residents' needs. Indirectly, this reflects well on the facility, which is important to the administration in terms of marketing. The social worker can stress this point when advocating for a strong residents' council.

CURRENT EVENTS GROUPS

Between my efforts and those of various staff members and volunteers, the current events group is held every weekday morning at the soldiers home. It was truly a product of the unique culture of the veterans' facility in that the ability to devote this amount of time to an ongoing group would be impossible if there

Figure 4. New York Yankees versus Boston Red Sox discussion in the current events group at the Soldiers' Home, 2008.

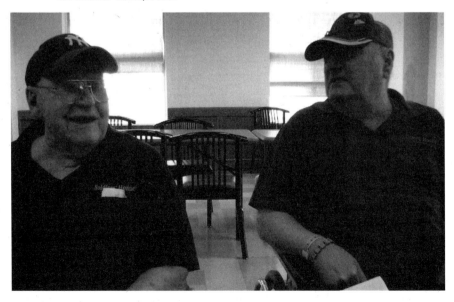

were additional mandatory meetings for the social worker to attend or if urgent discharge planning or other imperatives precluded setting aside a stretch of uninterrupted time for a daily residents' group. Even in the flexible, patient-oriented world where I worked, which valued the residents' well-being enough to support this group's continued existence, it was sometimes a juggling act to manage care-plan meetings, impromptu emergency situations, and the routine of a daily current events session. Nevertheless, I include this initiative and a description of the manner by which it was realized in the nursing home to show how a program can be developed to meet the psychosocial needs of residents perceived by the social worker and others, how such a program can be modified over time to address these needs better through ongoing assessment of its efficacy, and how even the initial goals of a particular program can shift as the endeavor evolves.

The current events group was four years old at the time of this writing. I started it when I observed that some of the more alert and oriented veterans appeared to be at loose ends after their morning ablutions were completed. There were not always activities scheduled, and when there were, they tended to reflect the typical morning routine that retired adults might follow, such as reading the paper or meeting with friends at the donut shop. As the staff social worker, I met with my director, as well as with the director of activities. We devised a joint plan to establish an informal coffee club in which those individuals who were able might come down from their rooms on their own to socialize. Coffee and newspapers, as well as cards and games, would be provided. We anticipated that the gathering would be able to function without a great deal of facilitation and agreed that we would take turns providing casual supervision at the site. Unfortunately, very few residents were able to negotiate the elevator to attend on their own, and, moreover, the residents required a good amount of encouragement (and enticement with doughnuts) before they were willing to come down at all. They did not understand the purpose of the program and tended to expect to be entertained once they got there.

The phenomenon of institutionalization has long been noted in individuals residing in long-term care facilities such as hospitals, nursing homes, and prisons, where there are limited opportunities for personal choices and everyone follows a rigidly routinized schedule. While such institutions were theoretically started for the benevolent reason of meeting the specialized needs of certain populations away from the mainstream of society (Wiersma, 2000), in fact, studies show that they engender behaviors of "learned helplessness and passivity" (Voelkl, 1985) in nursing home residents. Due to the negative effects of institutionalization and the not insignificant symptoms of depression, for which my population, frail older men, was at particular risk (Wolinsky, Callahan, Fitzgerald, & Johnson, 1992), the residents in the group initially appeared withdrawn, did not initiate conversations between themselves, and quickly became bored.

Clearly, more staff intervention was needed. How could we maintain the ambiance of an informal morning coffee hour while at the same time facilitating discussion about current events and meaningful interpersonal interactions? A routine for the sessions slowly evolved. At the suggestion of one resident, we made it our practice to read "This Day in History" ("It keeps your mind sharp," noted the resident) from the daily newspaper. Doing so generated a surprising amount of historical discussion. I was impressed (and remain so) with the veterans' grasp of American and world history, geography, and the basic sciences, the product, I believe, of an emphasis on memorization and factual information particular to their generation that in some ways is not matched in the education of subsequent eras. We also enjoyed reminiscing about events that occurred in the period of World War II. I made a special attempt to steer the conversation to such topics as rationing coupons, "old-time" medicinal remedies, Prohibition, their parents' immigration experiences, life during the Great Depression, the local burlesque district, the dance halls, music and entertainment of that era, and many other subjects. These subjects opened up quite a bit of discussion. In order to enhance the therapeutic value of these discussions, I made it a point to encourage the men to elaborate on the sensory details of the settings where the events being recounted took place to help them better access these memories, and I also focused on their relationships with others involved in these life events to help them process their feelings about these key people in their lives, as I described in the chapter on reminiscence and the life review. Talking about their common experiences growing up in the same era and locations tended to foster increased interaction and, over time, solidified quite a few friendships among the men. A few of the younger (Vietnam War–era) veterans were also able to bond around common experiences, and this has helped them feel less isolated, surrounded, as they were, by their older counterparts in the home.

In the beginning stages of the group, we were hesitant to include our less well-oriented residents, fearing that they might be disruptive or that the more functional participants would be "turned off" by the presence of their more mentally impaired cohorts, a not uncommon occurrence related to the fear of becoming, as if by contagion, "like them." However, when we did include other veterans who were seemingly quite disoriented, two things happened. The confused patients often exhibited very good long-term memories and social abilities that were not apparent in the ward setting, and the spirit of acceptance and camaraderie that prevailed in the group promoted a group norm of inclusiveness and tolerance. Thus, instead of simply meeting the needs of a privileged few, the current events group became a democratic forum open to all who could participate, with the exception of "wanderers," chiefly from the Alzheimer's unit, who could not be safely monitored in this setting.

In addition to the topics noted above, the group also enjoyed talking about sports, and this also became a regular part of the program. Gradually, we added such news events as scientific and astronomical discoveries. Curiously, they enjoyed having us read the obituaries of famous or locally well-known individuals and commenting upon these. It is with some sadness that I remember one of my favorite residents joking that he liked to check the obituaries to see if his name was present. He said he would be concerned if it was. He is dead now, but in his honor, the ritual of reading "This Day in History" and closing with the horoscope, both of which he had suggested, continues. Reading the horoscope works especially well as the closing ritual; it serves to acknowledge the existence of all members of the group, even if they did not actively participate in the session. The structure of the meeting was influenced greatly by this gentleman, and I like to think that it is to our credit that we were able to follow up on his good ideas.

As the current events group members and leaders became more comfortable with each other, we were able to discuss the war in Iraq and other unpleasant news items, and as a facilitator, I made great efforts to instill a spirit of the acceptance of differences of opinion about controversial subjects.

In terms of group leadership, quite a bit of perseverance on my part was essential in keeping this group running. I worked intensively with the activities director to secure volunteers to help out, sought and was granted permission to use unit secretaries as assistants at times, and finally obtained the services of a part-time activities professional. As I've noted before, I have found that, in general, co-leadership is much easier than running the group oneself. The presence of two facilitators adds greater dimension to the conversation and is helpful should the discussion lag. Moreover, it is helpful with transportation issues.

Since many of the men in the current events group are unable to come on their own, a significant part of making the arrangements for their transportation continued to be my responsibility. This was stressful at times but also brought secondary gains. It took a lot of work to gather the group together in the morning, paying special attention to encouraging new residents, as well as patients who appear withdrawn or who are in need of extra support to attend. However, in the process of making the transportation arrangements, I found myself doing informal rounds on the unit, chatting with residents and staff members, solving problems, and, just because I am on the spot, being privy to all sorts of resident-related issues that I probably would not have known about had I been less of a presence on the units. Still, it was my hope that as support for the program continued to grow in the facility, more assistants would be recruited, and my role in making transportation arrangements would decrease. This was desirable not only because the task is often quite tiring, but because it would be preferable that the project be less dependent on one person, thus insuring its future longevity.

SOME GENERAL METHODS

While the act of engaging seniors in reminiscence is at the core of bearing witness to and supporting the residents' individual identities and therefore figures prominently as a part of almost all of the programs that I have described, the goals of many of these undertakings have to do with particular needs of the population, such as adjustment to illness or increased socialization and sense of community, and therefore, in these situations, reminiscence is only one part of the agenda.

The quote at the beginning of this chapter making reference to the fact that in our present system of care we tend to think about and document our residents' personal attributes in an impersonal way demonstrates the conundrum of the facility (including the social worker) trying to meet the residents' individual needs with only limited knowledge of who these residents are. Undoubtedly, each resident's unique needs can be met only if the staff members first develop a relationship with the residents that enables them to get to know their patients as individuals. Certainly having the administration adopt structural changes that make the facility appear more homelike—providing on-site child care that integrates the community into the nursing home, creating a new family room with natural light, armchairs, and sofas, or adopting other practices associated with what Beth Baker (2007) calls "transformative" nursing homes—would be beneficial to the residents. However, because the likelihood of this spontaneously occurring on a large scale is negligible at this time, as I've argued throughout, social workers need to work from the bottom up to effect culture change. Resident-centered programs are one practical way to help begin this process.

While there is no recipe for the sorts of programs I have described, there are some general methods of approach to their development. Be aware of the needs of the particular population and define the goal or goals of the group accordingly. Ideally, the goals should be realistic and measurable. Devise a plan to meet those goals, focusing on the type of group, the estimated number of sessions the group will meet, and co-leadership (if any), among other things. Think through the overall structure of the sessions, including speakers, if any, and the sort of topics to be discussed. Then develop a tentative format for the sessions similar to a teacher's lesson plan: what will be discussed and the order of discussion, for example. Have a clear idea of the types of interventions you will focus on to meet therapeutic goals most effectively, for example, processing feelings of loss, empathizing and supporting others in the group, encouraging positive coping, encouraging individuals and the group to brainstorm about solutions to members' problems, or developing a culture of respect and caring in the group. Carefully plan out the logistics of the meetings—when and where the meetings will be held (a consistent time and place), how the residents will get to the group, whether there will be refreshments and how they will be supplied, and so on. Finally, develop a method for measuring the success of the group. For example, decreased depression might be measured by comparing the group members' scores on the Geriatric Depression Scale before the first meeting, midgroup, and after termination of the group (Sheikh & Yesavage, 1986; Yesavage, Brink, Rose, Lum, Huang, Adey, & Leirer, 1983). The observations of family and staff members, as well as data about the residents from the MDS, can also be indications of the group's effectiveness. Keep attendance records, your process notes, and notes of your own observations for future review, as well as for the purpose of project evaluation.

That being said, these types of programs tend to grow organically, their form and direction determined by a many factors, including the time and staff resources available, the support of the facility, the needs of the clients, and the skills and inclinations of the clinician.

Each morning, as I prepare to help gather the chair-bound residents from the various nursing units for "Current Events," I observe the residents who are able to wheel themselves into the activity room helping themselves to coffee and beginning to chat over the morning paper in anticipation of our morning ritual, and I realize that the reward for the social worker for persevering in the sometimes tiring effort of maintaining such a project is the joyful experience of the movement away from rigid institutional roles toward more authentic relationships between residents, as well as witnessing the sense of belonging that such programs confer on their participants.

Notes

1. In preparation for beginning a new group, I find it helpful to do an Internet search to familiarize myself with the topic at hand and to find out about organizations that might be able provide speakers as well as written information on developing a specialized support group for the condition in question. A Web search on the topic of "national stroke associations" provided the following:

The American Stroke Association (a division of the American Heart Association), National Center, 7272 Greenville Avenue, Dallas TX 75231; phone, AHA: 1-800-AHA-USA-1 (1-800-242-8721) or ASA: 1-888-4-STROKE (1-888-478-7653); Web site: www.strokeassociation.org. The American Stroke Association offers many programs and services, as well as links to local chapters.

The National Stroke Association, 9707 E. Easter Lane, Centennial, CO 80112; phone, 1-800-STROKES (1-800-787-6537); Web site: www.stroke.org. The National Stroke Association offers information on strokes, stroke prevention, stroke recovery, and stroke care. The Web site links to local chapters. A Web search for: "stroke organizations in [your state]" would give you even more specific information about local resources available to you.

2. National resources for the blind can be found at the American Federation for the Blind, online at www.afb.org. This site contains lots of information about living with vision loss and links to local service organizations and support groups.

Enrichment Audio Resource Services: Ears for Eyes Program (E.A.R.S) is a nonprofit organization providing free audiocassette tapes that teach adaptive living skills to the blind and their caregivers for seniors. They have a link that provides information about local support groups in each state. They can be reached at 1-800-843-6816 and on the Web at www.earsforeyes.org.

The National Federation of the Blind offers information about advocacy, education, research, technology, and programs encouraging independence. They can be reached at 1800 Johnson Street, Baltimore, MD 21230; phone (410) 659-9314; www.nfb.org. The Web site also has links to state and local organizations.

The Blinded Veterans Association offers resources for blind veterans. They can be reached at 447 H Street NW, Washington, D.C., 20001-2694; phone (202) 471-8880; www.bva.org.

Chapter 6

Programs for Staff

DESPITE THE BEST INTENTIONS OF SOCIAL WORKERS, NURSING HOME staff members, and administrators, and despite strict regulations, resident neglect or even mistreatment can occur, even in "good" nursing homes. As I've noted before, because long-term care facilities are financially driven, a corporate ethos can at times prevail. This can affect workers' ability to relate to their patients as human beings, rather than as tasks, and can negatively affect the provision of resident-focused care. In this chapter, I will show how we, as social workers, can have an effect on nursing home culture by promoting empathy and better staff-resident interactions. One of the ways we can do this is by working with the staff. Social workers can develop a role in staff education that will promote these objectives. One-hour in-service (on-the-job) training sessions are a good way to get started. Sensitivity training, which is like CPR for staff empathy, is one example of how social workers can work collaboratively with other staff members to promote resident-centered care.

Programs with staff members run by social workers don't generally work without the authorization by and participation from the nursing department, due to the social worker's role as an adjunct professional in this milieu. Once the social worker has participated in staff development programs, she can expand on this role by working collaboratively with outside services, such as a hospice or the facility's geriatric psychiatry team.

In the nursing home, nurses, doctors, and therapists each bring to the table their own particular professional perspectives on what it means to care for the residents. As Julie Abramson (2002) points out, each team member has already been socialized in his or her respective area of expertise. These professionals, along with the dietician, activities director, and social worker, constitute the interdisciplinary team. Clearly, in nursing homes, where the medical model prevails with its emphasis on physical needs and a problem-focused approach to care, residents are viewed as sick people with physical problems, and the care-plan team are the "authorities" who address their needs. The backbone of the facility, the certified nursing assistants (CNAs), working without a huge amount of formal training under the auspices of the nursing department, provide the routine care of making sure that the residents' day-to-day, minute-by-minute needs are met. These are the people who affect the residents' lives the most because they have the most contact with the residents and because the residents are dependent on them for almost every aspect of their daily existence.

CNAs are generally compassionate people who went into this line of work because they like helping others. Nursing assistants I have known have told me that their greatest joys involve providing this care to the best of their abilities and having positive relationships with the residents. Some of their greatest sorrows are losing a resident to death and seeing a resident suffer from the lack of a family support system, particularly on what are supposed to be festive occasions, such as birthdays and holidays. In a benign nursing home setting, there are enough positive aspects to their jobs to offset some of their greatest work-related challenges: dealing with verbal and/or physical abuse that residents may engage in due to, for example, changes in their mental status. The stresses of this job are many. CNAs are the among the most poorly compensated at the facility, and their position is not recognized as important in terms of formal status. The work is arduous and unremitting. What happens to the residents in situations where the training and support is not there for the caregivers?

To be a nurse is a critical responsibility. It is often said that while a doctor cures, a nurse heals. The skills involved in healing are many and demanding. A nurse's job requires accuracy and attention to detail. An error can mean the difference between life and death for their patients. Doctors regularly depend on their skills in making assessments and treatment decisions. Nurses must be able to educate patients about their illnesses, comfort and reassure them, deal with their behavior and their emotional concerns, provide support to their families, and much, much more. In addition to these responsibilities, they must lead their staff with a skillful combination of "tough love" and nurturance or else their directives will surely be met with a measure of hostility and resistance. What happens to the residents when the administration, pressed to meet the financial requirements of the institution and objective standards of quality of care set out by the regulations, neglects to be responsive to the needs of those on whose healing presence the residents depend?

What can happen in these situations is that the emotional needs of residents will surely go by the wayside. This can occur insidiously. Staff members, including social workers, may not even realize this is happening, so caught up are they in the daily routine of their jobs. What happens is that the inevitable stress of endlessly giving of oneself to an incessantly needy population, with the added stress of coping with death and loss on a routine basis and the focus on human beings as bodies rather than people, may lead us to forget to be mindful of what it feels like to be on "the other side of the bedpan," as Elizabeth Downton (2007), a geriatric social worker, put it in an essay written when she found herself in the role of a patient at a nursing care facility for rehabilitation following surgery:

> I was afraid to leave the hospital because I felt safe there. The nurses and doctors at the hospital were very kind. They kept me until Friday. I can't praise the hospital staff enough. I could not bend to wipe myself, and they made it seem that doing this was normal and part of their jobs.
>
> The degradation began when I was transferred to a recuperative and long-term care center. Friday afternoon, I arrived at rehab desperately needing to urinate. It took forever for them to put me in a room and for someone to help me to the toilet. After allowing me to urinate, the staff weighed me and announced my weight to the world (the staff there and the two other occupants of the room). They said that I was over the weight limit by a few pounds. This was very embarrassing, because I had struggled with my weight for years and was extremely sensitive about it. Immediately, I noticed differences in the level of care from what I had received in the hospital. Those first few days, I had to use the bathroom frequently. Although I was not allowed to get out of bed alone, I often had to. When I rang for help, it often took half an hour or more. Furthermore, unless I had a bowel movement, I stopped requesting assistance wiping myself after I heard the aides arguing in the hallway over who would help me off the toilet and wipe me. ("You go; I ain't going.") You can imagine how this made me feel. I was mortified and intimidated at the same time. After all, I was at the mercy of these people. I can hardly imagine how a terminal or dementia patient feels. This is supposedly one of the better recuperative centers.

Even in the best facilities, when the culture of the institution is one of corporate efficiency rather than one of caring, as in the above account, the result is that, while the staff may ostensibly be doing their jobs, to the patient they can appear to be both physically and emotionally absent. This includes the social worker. When I asked the author of this sad commentary where the social worker was throughout her ordeal, she noted with some surprise that she did not remember seeing one or, if she did, the interview did not stand out in her mind. The fact that the very individual who could have interceded on her behalf seems to be inexplicably missing from the scene in this account—by someone who is herself a geriatric social worker—is something that all of us should take under advisement when we think we are too busy to do more than the necessary paperwork, attending by this paper compliance to the letter rather than the spirit of our mandate. The values and mores of the culture in which we work can affect us all in insidious ways.

While by no means a statistical survey of the average nursing home rehabilitation experience, this essay is a sadly realistic commentary about what can happen to caring, dedicated professionals and paraprofessionals who started out with every intention of doing their jobs well. As social workers, we can recognize and evaluate the effect of this aspect of our environment on ourselves and others and ultimately work toward reversing the negative spiral of disaffected workers and poor care that is a constant risk in an institutional environment.

SENSITIVITY TRAINING IN GROUPS: EMERGENCY RESUSCITATION FOR EMPATHY

Hearing this social work colleague relate her experience as a patient in a professional workshop served as a mini wake-up call to conference participants. Undoubtedly we had all heard similar complaints before about residents waiting too long to be taken to the bathroom. However, when the plaintiff was not a debilitated, marginalized elder but a peer, suddenly we listened with new ears. The surprising revelation that this could be me brought with it the visceral realization that not only are our residents being treated in an impersonal manner, but also that they are viewed by their caregivers as something less than fully sentient human beings. This "Aha" moment brought us all closer to empathizing with our clients' experiences and emphasized for me the fact that there is a clear need for a major attitude change: ours.

One of the methods at our disposal for helping staff to remember their professional mission is sensitivity training. Indeed, the promotion of such epiphanies is the essence of sensitivity training. To do this, social workers can use their creativity to raise coworkers' awareness of the disconnect that may exist between their intentions and their actions. While sensitivity training is perceptibly needed in nursing homes, however, it is not often performed there. Of course, resident neglect and abuse are decried by the administration. One reason for this is that the facility will be sanctioned by the department of public health for such occurrences. When this happens, blame often ensues, and the "guilty party" is disciplined. Thus, the very positive benefits of facility oversight by the government ushered in by the Nursing Home Reform Act are ironically offset by the rigidity of the manner in which they may be at times enforced, resulting in a perceived adversarial relationship between state surveyors and nursing home administrators (Stafford, 2003). The negativity generated by this method of avoiding bad care often seems to supersede an attitude of genuine concern for the residents' welfare (McLean, 1997).

While mulling over these dilemmas, I attended a nursing home conference where I had the good fortune of sitting next to Beverly Noiseau, a very competent and seasoned social work colleague who had done extensive work in the area of sensitivity training. We struck up a conversation, and she told me about some very exciting workshops that she had developed to improve staff interactions with residents. She performed one of her training programs at my facility, and I have been using variations of her program ever since with excellent results.

The basic concept behind these workshops for frontline care-giving staff is an abrupt role reversal. In short order, like Elizabeth Downton on "the other side of the bedpan," trainees are stripped of their former identities, their physical independence, and their dignity and subjected to the vicissitudes of having their physical and emotional needs "met" by trainers playing the role of indifferent, thoughtless, and uncaring attendants. In doing so, they gain a very real understanding that to be a handicapped, helpless, and dependent resident in this situation is to feel, as a new worker in my agency who participated in such a role play described with tears in her eyes, "as if I am nothing."

This type of role playing, I am told by my nursing colleagues, is often employed with nurse-trainees in schools of nursing, but unfortunately it is rarely reviewed in actual work settings. I have, incidentally, never heard of it being used in social work teaching situations. Despite the great focus on awareness of ethnic and social diversity in college and work settings, social workers are not often challenged to consider the emotional ramifications of medical conditions affecting client's physical and cognitive abilities.

The beauty of my colleague's program is its elegant simplicity. Her methods include providing subjects with glasses smeared with Vaseline to simulate low vision, stuffing earplugs in their ears to mimic deafness, and securing their arms to give participants an idea of what it is like to be paralyzed by a stroke. Placed in wheelchairs, the workshop participants are treated to an intentionally harsh version of care by the facilitators. This may include being placed in a wheelchair and transported abruptly, without advance warning. It may also involve trying to eat a meal without the use of one's dominant hand or the frustration of being fed in a rushed and unsolicitous manner. The workshop also generally includes the experience of hearing others laughingly address each other in a (real or imaginary) language that the subject does not understand or of being ignored while their caregivers discuss their personal lives among themselves. All of this, of course, is intended to simulate some of the situations nursing home residents may experience during such activities as mealtime or other aspects of their daily routine.

After the experiential portion of the training is completed, participants have the chance to process their emotions and, having walked a mile in their shoes, to empathize with those who must permanently endure the handicaps of blindness, hearing loss, and loss of mobility that trainees have momentarily experienced. I have found that an important aspect of the debriefing process is that it take place in an atmosphere of caring, humor, and support. It can actually be quite fun for everybody, and much laughter may ensue. This training must not be used as a way of shaming or blaming staff for their behavior but instead should be used to model a caring, "we are all in this together" mindset.

In my own work, I have been fortunate enough to have the support of a very committed nurse manager, Linda, who is able to see both the details and the big picture of her patients' needs. Linda and I have worked together on a variety of programs, including conducting sensitivity training workshops for new nurses and nursing assistants as part of their orientation process. It is extremely helpful work with her as a co-leader in these sessions because of her firsthand knowledge and understanding of nursing staff and the work that they do.

Sensitivity Training Sessions for New Staff

The sessions that we use to train new staff members last about an hour and stress the importance of considering the residents' physical limitations and their need for attentive care and emotional support in an atmosphere of inclusiveness. In addition, they point out the important function that staff members can have in helping to restore the residents' sense of identity which was lost when they acquired their new role as patients. The format of the sessions is as follows.

1) Introductions (5 to 10 minutes)

Co-leaders introduce themselves, then go around the room asking new workers to do the same and to report a little bit about their backgrounds and why they became certified nursing assistants or nurses. In our sessions, I work with the nurse manager to raise new staff members' consciousness about the importance of considering the residents' physical limitations and being aware of the residents' feelings. The sessions last about an hour to an hour and a half. No residents are present, because we hold frank discussions that would compromise patient confidentiality. We strive to create a safe place for staff to express their thoughts and emotions, and in so doing try to model for staff members the emotional support and inclusiveness that we hope they will bring to their interactions with the residents.

2) Definition and discussion of the meaning of sensitivity as it relates to the work at hand (10 to 15 minutes)

Sensitivity is generally defined as an awareness of the needs and feelings of other people. Participants can be asked to give examples of sensitive and insensitive behavior toward residents, and leaders can initiate a discussion of these examples. Leaders may also wish to discuss reasons why workers might not be sensitive at certain times due to stress, fatigue, or prejudices. Self-awareness with regard to one's cultural and ethnic beliefs should be encouraged. This section can be tailored to the needs of participating groups. For instance, in a session with new nursing school graduates who had formerly been nursing assistants at the facility, Linda chose to focus on issues of leadership that the nurses need to be aware of and sensitive to, such as the change in their role and its effect on the staff that they will be supervising. In this case, the new workers were encouraged to be sensitive and respectful to the staff, yet firm in their expectations of them due to the responsibility of the nursing role.

3) Role playing (about 10 to 15 minutes)

Leaders use prepared props to turn the trainees into "residents" (for example, Vaseline-smeared glasses, earplugs, scarves to bind hands to simulate the effects of paralysis), then serve crackers, juice, or other snacks to simulate mealtime while conversing together about inappropriate topics (for example, personal life, "Can't wait to get out of here," other residents, the residents' bowel movements) in English or in a foreign language, totally ignoring the residents.

4) Discussion of the role playing (10 to 15 minutes)

It is important to help staff members process their feelings about the experience of being a helpless and impaired "resident" at the mercy of an uncaring staff. Generally, this is experienced as very painful. Leaders can solicit participants' observations of what they did wrong as pretend staff members, and the group can talk about better approaches to resident care. At this point, I like to encourage staff members to relate to their charges in a caring and professional manner by selectively sharing personal (but not intimate) information that may be indicated by the conversation, to the extent that staff members feel comfortable doing so. This may include anecdotes about their own childhood, their children, or about their own lives. The focus here is the goal of bonding with and better understanding the residents, as opposed to chatting with their friends at work as in the role playing or burdening the residents with their own difficulties.

The staff members tend to be relieved to be released from the feelings of isolation and helplessness engendered by the role playing and energized and enlightened by the experience, and I have noticed that at this point they are usually very receptive to suggestions of improved approaches to resident care. I have also observed that new employees who have received an orientation that included this training tend to maintain a positive attitude toward their work and an understanding of the importance of their role in the residents' lives and well-being.

5) Further role playing related to participants' concerns (5 to 10 minutes)

If time permits, staff members and residents can act out difficult situations that they will encounter in the course of their jobs, such as verbal or physical abuse by agitated residents, demanding behavior by emotionally needy residents, or multiple demands at once from many residents. When these exercises are processed by the participants, the group can be asked to do problem-solving exercises and come up with solutions to these dilemmas. Linda always encourages new staff members to ask for help from their supervisor if they feel unsure of themselves.

6) Wrap-up (5 minutes)

Leaders summarize the meeting, solicit group feedback, validate the participation of staff members and their insights, provide support and encouragement about the staff members' ability to perform well and to be sensitive to the residents, and offer to be available for consultation about questions related to this topic in the future.

Expanding on This Beginning

After observing that the effects of our programs were well understood and accepted by new trainees but that the effects of sensitivity training tended to wear off as the new workers assimilated into the culture of the facility, the nursing administrator decided to adapt the format of our group sessions for new employees into an ongoing sensitivity in-service training for all staff, particularly for those who had been observed to require increased sensitivity in their interactions with residents or families. For instance, several caregivers were referred after family members heard them complain as they performed post-mortem care that the body of a deceased resident was "heavy."

Our program is now held monthly for a two-hour block of time with a rotating group of four to six staff members who are mandated to attend. The content of the sessions is generally geared to issues that the staff members may be having, such as the one just mentioned regarding death and bereavement. On another occasion, we engaged a guest speaker from a local gay, bisexual, lesbian, and transgender elder advocacy group to address staff members who were noted to be discussing homosexuality at the bedside of a resident whose son was gay. We worked with the director of this organization to help staff members feel less threatened by those with alternative sexual orientations and to perceive them as people, rather than as stereotypes. By the end of an interactive discussion in a safe setting, group members came to the conclusion that "people are just people" and resolved to set an example by refraining from joining any homophobic conversations in which their peers engaged.

STAFF TRAINING AND CULTURE CHANGE

Role reversal is an excellent tool for raising staff members' consciousness about the necessity of connecting with and listening to the residents. It addresses the tendency of staff members to assign little importance to their charges or their job. The unfortunate situation of disengaged and indifferent staff members is a risk in any facility, just because it is a place of business, for-profit or not, and as such (especially in the case of for-profit situations) presents a conflict of interest for those working there. As Philip Stafford (2003) trenchantly observes, the fact that the nursing home is a culturally ambiguous place may be its most problematic feature. It is at once a total institution and a medicalized environment that strives to achieve a homelike atmosphere. The staff members working in such places are caring people, caring for people, and in many ways, serving in the role of surrogate family for the residents. At the same time, the work that they do in the nursing home is their job and their livelihood, and they are working for administrators who want to make a profit. Is it any small wonder that staff members can get caught up and become frustrated by the conflicting pressures to meet their own needs, to meet the residents' needs, and to fulfill the requirements of their job descriptions to the satisfaction of their employers?

Finding a balance is hard. The social worker can have a role in engaging others to work toward aligning the facility's goals of better patient outcomes and more effective use of staff time with the professional goals and values of the staff. One of the ways she can do this is by imaginative use of staff education that promotes a culture of caring. A culture of caring is in everyone's interest—staff, residents, and administrators alike. CNAs, in particular, have been found to work better when they are engaged, valued, and respected as team members (Yeatts & Cready, 2007). Thus, by participating in staff development activities, the social worker can facilitate conflict resolution between the corporate administration and the staff. Despite their differences, administrators and staff members have certain negotiable concerns and definite areas of common interest. Administrators would like a cooperative, committed workforce. Staff members would like a caring, responsive workplace whose values are in line with their professional values. Both would like to uphold the best interests of the residents. The social worker can promote a focus on this common objective.

By applying social work principles through the use of social work skills, we can have a positive effect on our environment. Working with staff members and the administration, we can remind others of the importance of the residents' holistic needs and make a contribution that can result in a more resident-centered focus of care that will not only positively affect resident well-being but may improve staff members' attitudes and the facility's financial profit as well.

PROGRAMS FOR STAFF MEMBERS THAT DIDN'T WORK AND WHY

Not all educational training provided by social workers will necessarily accomplish the sought-after systemwide changes in attitudes and values described above. The programs must generally be performed in collaboration with the nursing department, because the nursing home is run and operated by nurses. Without nursing administrative approval and input from someone at the nurse management level or higher, a staff education initiative aimed at nursing and CNAs will have little lasting influence on the participants. This makes sense because the social worker is a collateral staff member in the nursing home setting.

Early in my career, I attempted to run a support group for certified nursing assistants. I felt that the staff members where I was then employed were unhappy and underappreciated. I wished to support them and hoped to encourage them to support one another's efforts and achievements in dealing with challenging situations and maintaining an attitude of compassion toward the residents, even when such positive achievements were not recognized or rewarded by their superiors. This goal was met with moderate success, in that the workers expressed that they liked me, and I quite admired them. However, in terms of having an actual effect on patient care, I doubt that the group was tremendously helpful for a variety of reasons.

First, in focusing primarily on the needs of CNAs, the emphasis on patient care tended to be lost, and the meetings often degenerated into gripe sessions with little that I could do as the facility social worker to address the grievances. Also, I did this project on my own, with no facility collaboration (except, of course, for the administrator's permission). Due to my outsider status in terms of the facility, I had no authority to make changes for the workers, to help them to feel integrated into the fabric of the facility, or to advocate strongly for the needs of the residents. I would not perform such a group again unless I worked closely with nursing administration in planning and running the meetings.

DEVELOPING THE SOCIAL SERVICE ROLE IN PROGRAM DEVELOPMENT FOR STAFF MEMBERS

As the saying goes, a journey begins with a single step, and the same is true of developing a social work role in the area of staff education. Some of the earliest educational activities that I attempted with staff members have been in the form of short in-service training sessions, rather than an ongoing program. Presentations about resident rights and resident abuse have long been part of the nursing home social worker's job. Although these are mandated and endorsed by the administration, reading from a prepared speech is the usual way we are expected to discharge this responsibility. To get away from this particular standard, I tried to infuse some creativity into the process of performing social service staff training. Instead of merely going over a list of resident rights or listing the various forms of potential abuse, I worked with my colleagues to act out scenarios where residents were depicted as being inappropriately treated. In one of these vignettes, a staff member playing a resident sat in a wheelchair and was approached from behind without warning and abruptly pushed to the dining room. This role playing was followed by discussions of what constituted resident abuse and why. In the above example, we talked about how the resident was not treated with dignity, was not given a choice about being taken to supper, and was emotionally abused by being frightened by someone with more power than she had. Other scenarios depicted a frustrated staff member striking a resident and a staff member opening a resident's mail without permission. The staff developer filmed our presentation, and as a result, not only the participants, but staff members on other shifts enjoyed seeing what was for most of them familiar information being presented in a new way, one that had a greater potential for being effective due to its use of an experiential format.

Running single in-service training sessions such as this taught me much about working with other nursing home staff. From this foray into the area of teaching at my facility, I learned the importance of finding a way to work with the different disciplines to meet the residents' psychosocial needs by developing a common language in which to discuss the areas of overlap between our professional objectives. I also applied what I already knew about the need to work closely with other departments, particularly nursing, to format my teachings in such a way that they would be accepted by the facility. Unlike my first attempt at staff program development with CNAs, I was not working as a Lone Ranger. However, despite the fact that I had involved the staff developer in planning the program, I actually implemented it by myself, and that, I now appreciated, was what condemned the training to remain outside of the accepted practice of the facility.

This was the lesson I had in mind when I worked in partnership with the nursing department in the area of sensitivity training. It was also something I kept in mind when I expanded my teaching activities to include working with other human service agencies affiliated with the facility to provide specialized educational programming for facility employees. However, one does not need anything so elaborate as a video camera to present a single in-service training session. These can be developed and presented in a straightforward manner that both meets the social worker's mandated requirements and addresses staff-related social service concerns that the social worker may perceive at her facility. For instance, I noticed at one point that I was observing (and participating in) discussions where staff members expressed frustration with family members who were perceived very much as outsiders in a "them versus us" struggle over the residents' care. At these times, I was rather unpleasantly surprised to hear myself agreeing with and even making disapproving remarks about the way in which family members coped with their loved one's being in a nursing home, especially when their coping methods included seemingly endless and unrealistic complaints about that resident's care to staff members, administrators, and whoever else would listen. "So and so is such a pain," we would say. "It's unrealistic that she wants her mother up and dressed in her best clothes and neat as a pin no matter what time she comes in. The one time Mrs. Green had food on her clothes from lunch, the daughter went and filed a complaint about it!" After some reflection on my own attitudes and beliefs concerning difficult family members, I realized that while part of me identified with the staff's annoyance at these "interlopers" who were "interfering" with our daily routine, my ingrained professional training informed me that not only are there two sides to the story, but that family members are an essential part of the residents' support network and as such help to ensure the residents' well-being.

To address this problem, I designed a brief in-service session that would help staff members communicate better with family members. It used the elements of lecture, discussion, and role playing to convey the concepts of building trust with family members, identifying family strengths, and working with these strengths to improve patient outcomes. It culminated with a mock "family meeting" in which staff members played the roles of resident, interdisciplinary team, and family members working to develop common care-plan goals based the resident's and family's understanding of the resident's situation and to design care-plan interventions based the strengths of the resident and family. The presentation helped staff members to understand that confrontations with family members such as the one described above can be minimized when we, as caregivers, take the time to build solid, respectful relationships with family members. The program was well received, and participation was enthusiastic. Not only did the experience of presenting this program help me in developing skill and confidence as a teacher, but the research that I did in preparing my presentation helped me both expand my knowledge and consolidate my ideas about the role of the social worker in the nursing home.

WORKING WITH OUTSIDE SERVICES

Outside service providers generally play a large role in providing social services in today's nursing homes. Hospice programs, which provide services for the terminally ill in their homes, are also contracted by nursing homes to assist with the pain management and care needs of residents with a diagnosis of six months or less to live. They bring with them additional social services to counsel the patients and their families, as well as spiritual services in the form of an ecumenical minister. In addition, many nursing homes obtain geriatric psychiatric services from companies providing these in the form of a comprehensive mental health team composed of social workers, psychiatric nurse practitioners, psychologists, and psychiatrists who visit the facility and offer behavioral interventions, individual counseling, and psychiatric medication management. Both of these services complement the work done by the facility social worker on the premises (although I have often felt that more facility social service hours, with an emphasis on group therapy and the existence of meaningful psychosocial programming, would lessen the need for psychiatric services for residents).

Given the reality of the current social service staff time available, the staff social worker can enhance her productivity by developing relationships with the staff of these service providers, working collaboratively with them, and staff education is an important way in which we can collaborate.

When working with outside resources to present staff training programs, it is always advantageous to involve facility staff members in the process. Asked to present a program with our hospice service on grief and bereavement, I immediately discussed the project with the unit managers with whom I work in order to solicit their input. As a result of our discussion, we arranged to weave the program around a particular case that had involved both of us. The case involved a resident we felt would benefit from hospice services for support concerning her imminent death, but her family was reluctant to have these services and the staff perceived the family to have persuaded the resident to decline hospice care, as well. As we discussed our feelings of sadness and frustration at this situation, we came as a group to a better understanding of the family's concerns, as well as of our need to engage this family, who were clearly experiencing difficulty accepting and coping with their anticipatory grief. The training was thus significantly different and more tailored to our specific needs than it would have been had the hospice simply presented a generic program from their training manual.

LENDING A HAND

In the nursing home, we do not often serve in the role of an employee assistance social worker for nursing home staff members, but as social workers we can make ourselves available to help staff members find resources for child care, housing, or education, or refer them to agencies that can help them deal with these and other issues of concern. This assistance not only benefits the staff members themselves but also indirectly helps the residents for whom they care, as it will decrease the stress that the caregivers experience. It goes without saying that when assisting coworkers with these matters, their confidentiality should be respected at all times.

Carving out a social work role in the area of staff development takes time and persistence. One way to get started might be to experiment with presenting short in-service training sessions. Using our skills to educate other workers not only helps to make a difference in our residents' lives but provides us with an exciting opportunity for personal and professional growth.

Chapter 7

Programs for Families

SO FAR, WE HAVE DISCUSSED PROGRAMMATIC INTERVENTIONS WITH RESidents and staff as components of the residents' support network. We now turn to another highly important component of our residents' lives: their families. While these individuals no longer provide direct care to their loved ones as they may have done before, their continued involvement, in as positive a manner as possible, is crucial to the residents' well-being. (Indeed, residents who lack families or who are estranged from their relatives require special social work care and attention in order to reestablish ties or to try to compensate by developing other sustaining ties).

Social workers need to remember to be mindful of the fact that what is a routine occurrence in her world is almost always an emotionally devastating event for everyone involved in the family constellation. The decision to place someone is most often made when there are no other options left. Relatives often struggle for years with the burdens of caregiving until they are too exhausted, both emotionally and physically, to do so any longer. Frequently, it is a health crisis for the caregiver that ultimately precipitates the resident's need for placement in a nursing home.

The social worker's role with families of newly admitted residents is to provide lots and lots of reassurance that their ambivalent feelings of guilt mixed with relief are normal. Added to this mixture is a measure of shame. Faith Gibson (2004) states: "Admission to a residential care facility from a family base is a public declaration that the caregiver has failed in a job, either willingly or reluctantly attempted" (p. 251). In fact, families' secret feelings of self-blame are unjustified. No matter how someone may have promised in the past never to place a loved one in a nursing home, circumstances will have changed since that guarantee was made. Despite all of the family's often amazingly valiant efforts, at this point, their relative's care needs as perceived and experienced by the family will have become too great for them to manage with the limited services available in the community. We can anticipate that many family members will experience feelings of guilt, even though they may have been jeopardizing their own physical and mental health in their efforts to provide care at home. We can provide support and reassurance to families, for instance, by point out that the family members are of no help to their loved one if they do not care for themselves and become sick.

The nursing home social worker can also assure families that their caregiving role need not end because their loved one is now in a nursing home. Depending on the facility, the family, if they wish, can still provide a limited amount of hands-on care, for example, assisting with the resident's grooming or helping to feed the resident a meal, by making arrangements with the nurse unit manager. Most importantly, the social worker should always stress the great emotional benefits that residents derive from family contact and family visits.

Social workers in their individual work with family members can and should play a role in helping them to enjoy positive visits with their loved ones. Depending on the domestic situation and the resident, there may be an initial period of adjustment for a few weeks, a time in which the family refrains from frequent contact in order to avoid interactions that are distressing to both the resident and themselves as they all adjust to the reality of separation. (This is particularly true in the case where the resident has dementia and is unable to understand and process the situation fully.) However, in the end, residents and families can achieve closeness and connectedness that may have been lost in the daily struggle to maintain a frail dependent elder who, due to disease, may no longer have been in control of his or her actions or behavior.

Suggestions for visits depend on the social worker's knowledge of the individual resident and family. In most cases, both the resident and the family will benefit from being reminded of the resident's identity in happier and more independent times, and having the family bring in old photos and albums to peruse with their loved one is most appropriate. If the resident had a beloved pet, arrangements can often be made with the facility for the animal to be brought in to visit, which provides inestimable comfort to the resident. Books or items related to the resident's hobbies and interests can be brought in (for example, stamp or coin collections, books about travel, sailing, or art, crochet hook and yarn if the resident is still able to use it). Games such as checkers, cards, and cribbage can be played with the resident, and providing a resident with these items can lead to their finding new friends to share these activities when the family is not there. Family photos or a small compact disc player with a selection of cherished music can be brought in to share with the resident, and arrangements can be made for the staff to help make these items available to the resident to remind them of their family's love when the family is not there. In this vein,

Figure 5. Resident and family members discussing resident's past accomplishments at a care-plan meeting.

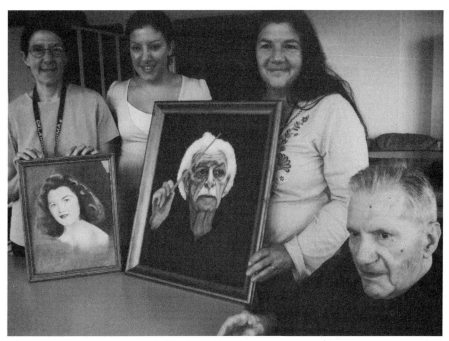

recordings of the family reminiscing about happy events involving the resident can sometimes be used as transitional objects to help the resident cope with the separation from his or her family, particularly if the resident is confused due to dementia.

Often, generally after the resident has made an adjustment to the facility, outings with family members are possible, and the care-plan team, with the assistance of the social worker, can help the family make transportation arrangements for the resident to visit with the family at a restaurant, in the family home, or at a location of their choice. It is best to follow the resident's and family's lead in arranging resident outings with family. Previous family dynamics of which we are not always aware play an important role in whether such outings are indicated. In one case, for example, during a discussion of the activity programs available at the facility in an early interdisciplinary meeting with a newly admitted resident and her son, the activities director reported that it was possible for family members to attend facility outings, such as trips to a baseball game or the shopping mall. I wondered why the son did not bring up the issue of bringing the resident to his home, which was nearby. Directly after the meeting, he disclosed that the relationship had been a difficult one and that his mother, who appeared to be sweet and good-natured, had been overly critical and bad-tempered when the son was growing up and had only changed after the onset of dementia. Understandably, the son had ambivalent feelings about his caregiving role.

Naturally, an adult child of a resident who may have been sexually abusive will probably not wish to take that resident home for a visit. On the other hand, a younger resident who is alert and oriented and her spouse may wish to have conjugal visits, and the social worker can sensitively work with the resident, family, and interdisciplinary team to arrange for this personal matter. The social worker should always work with the interdisciplinary team, and in particular with the unit nurse manager, in making arrangements for resident outings and advocating for the resident. Sharing her information on the family context with the team helps them to understand both the resident's and family's positions, and using the input of the team will help to make sure that the visits are safe and go smoothly.

Young children often have a difficult time coping with the sights and sounds of the nursing home, as well as with their discomfort at seeing their beloved grandparent or great-grandparent exhibit what appears to be, in our youth-oriented society, disfiguring and/or socially unacceptable disabilities and behaviors. Engaging the child in making a simple craft project with or for the elder, perhaps in the activity room, away from the chaos of a crowded unit, is a good way to help the child focus on relating to their relative, rather than observing the inevitable effects of time from an impersonal distance. Social workers should also make a point of letting families know that they can always make arrangements with the activities director or other designated facility contact to secure a room and assistance from the kitchen for family parties and celebrations, which can be a very upbeat intergenerational experience for family members.

In addition to all that the social worker can do individually to assist families with the transition to having their loved one in a nursing home and to maximize the benefits of family visits, it is important to empower families who wish to do so to be a part of the nursing home community and to have a say in its functioning. The primary way of doing this is through their participation in an active and effective family council.

THE FAMILY COUNCIL

A family council consists of a group of family members who meet regularly for the purpose of enhancing residents' care and their quality of life. Federal regulations strongly support the existence of family councils in nursing homes but fall short of actually requiring them unless family members specifically request one. If a family council does exist, the law is specific in its stipulations that the facility make adequate provisions for it, including a space to meet privately, a facility liaison to provide assistance to the group, and follow-up efforts on written requests that are generated by the meetings.

The family council is an important forum in which families can participate in the functioning of the nursing home. Family councils can enhance communication between staff members, residents, and families and thus improve the operation of nursing homes in significant ways, including improving employee efficiency and satisfaction. They also provide mutual support and empowerment for family members and a viable avenue for their continued involvement in their loved one's care. It is therefore axiomatic that we, as social workers, should advocate for the formation of family councils and work to help to facilitate the autonomous functioning of them, as the "voice of the families."

The family council at the soldiers' home is an example of a group that is fully integrated into the life of the facility. The council's involvement in facility policy and procedures is accepted as a given, and their views and opinions are regarded with a great deal of respect by all. The president of the council enjoys an open-door relationship with the commandant, who is the facility's chief administrator. Staff members are grateful for the holiday parties that the council sponsors on the units, as well as for the numerous other ways in which it recognizes employees' work and improves the lives of the residents. The council is also known for hosting bingo games for the residents and treating facility volunteers to an annual luncheon. The soldiers' home T-shirts, which the family council sells at its "yard sales" to raise money for its various projects, are an accepted part of the staff uniform, which demonstrates how closely the family council's identity is associated with that of the soldiers' home.

My former director of social services started this family council some time ago. When she undertook this project, she worked closely with the administration, engaging them in the process of implementing the program, an approach that resulted their high degree of investment in its success. This proved to be key to the council's effectiveness and longevity.

In working out the logistics of the council functioning, this director engaged the assistance of a colleague who had experience in starting and developing other family councils. On his advice, she adopted a structured format for her meetings that included having elected officers (a president, vice president, and secretary), adhering to regular meeting times, an agenda, and the adoption of Robert's Rules of Order. To this day, the council president bangs a gavel to bring the meetings to order, but it should be noted that she does so with humor and tact. In laying the groundwork for her program, the director worked with the council to write a mission statement, as well as by-laws, thus cementing the council's procedures into statutes. One of the procedures was (and continues to be) that the minutes taken by the council secretary are typed and mailed out to all families by clerical staff members at the facility. Another protocol that was later adopted involves the family council president maintaining an information column in the monthly facility newsletter. Finally, the director of social services put procedures into place stipulating that new families be made aware of the council, both through written material and by facility social workers as part of the family's orientation process. All of these measures, plus the provision of a very nice luncheon for the families at the monthly meetings, have ensured a consistently high attendance (usually about thirty people) over the past twenty years.

A major reason for this particular group's success and longevity is that family members were encouraged to have a great deal of autonomy in their meetings. Instead of facilitating the entire meeting, the director of social services, as facility liaison, makes an appearance only at the beginning, to convey announcements, and at the end, to check in with members about their concerns. Indeed, the National Citizens' Coalition for Nursing Home Reform (NCCNHR), a nonprofit organization founded in 1975 that represents at least two hundred grassroots advocacy groups nationwide, supports the concept of a family-led council, as opposed to one that is run by the facility with only nominal input from family members.[1] While autonomy is an ultimate goal for family councils, in many facilities, the current reality is that no family council exists or there is only a token one. These conditions require the social worker to take an active role in initiating the proceedings, such as my director did during the initial stages of council formation at the veterans' facility.

Having had the experience of starting family councils in other facilities, I am acutely aware of the distinct advantages that the family council at the soldiers' home enjoys in its ability to run a positive and effective forum. The experience of family council development in a private facility is different because of the inherent conflict of interest between a corporation with a for-profit motive, an institutional context that tends to cast family members in the role of consumers, and the families themselves, who are experiencing their role as caregivers being usurped by an institutional model of care. This disconnect is minimized at the soldiers' home, because the institution recognizes the contributions of the veterans it serves, thus unifying families and the facility's administration in a common mission toward the residents based on their identity and its agreed-upon social importance. I would expect that families and the administration share similar alliances in nursing homes that are dedicated to the care of those who were engaged in a particular vocation (for example, a mariners' home, or a home for retired priests) or even dedicated to a particular ethnic group (for example, a Chinese nursing home or a Jewish facility). Any kind of nonprofit operation would be more likely to have a charter that more closely aligns the goals of families with the goals of those who run the institution. However, because the for-profit corporate nursing home struggles to unite two disparate tasks—caring and making money—strained relationships often occur.

In the for-profit nursing home, the ambivalence and frustration that family members have about the need to place their loved one in long-term care tend to get played out more readily in a conflictual manner. In these cases, as I've noted before, families might perceive the facility as unresponsive and incompetent at such things as remembering the details of their loved one's personal preferences and individual care needs, while the facility might view the family members as unrealistic and overly critical of the care. Unfortunately, both perceptions are usually true. All of this is to point out that most nursing home social workers must deal with several challenging systemic issues when they start a family council or work to develop one that is already in place.

When a social worker wishes to start (or improve) a family council under these challenging circumstances, a primary task is to work with the administration to generate enthusiasm for the project. In doing so, the social worker might initially try to solicit the administrator's hopes for the council, as well any concerns that the administrator might have. Common goals can then be embraced, differences negotiated, and anticipated obstacles addressed. As an example of the latter, the administrator might express concern that the council could turn into a "gripe session," further escalating the anger of angry families. An actively engaged social worker, while agreeing that this is a possibility, could point out that satisfied families tend to be supportive of a facility and to help market it by word of mouth. Therefore, if the facility can build trust with the families by being responsive to the suggestions of a council and working together with them toward common goals, it is likely that positive dynamics in all of the facility's dealings with families will result. By thus allying herself with the administrator's position, the social worker can improve her chances of turning the discussion into a constructive, problem-solving one instead of falling into the trap of getting into a struggle based on the different agendas of the social services department and the administration. Even if the initial discussion with the administrator does not go well, the social worker has set the stage for further discussions about collaborative efforts to engage families, which may in turn result in successful projects that ultimately pave the way for the existence of a formal council.

If the administration agrees to develop a family council, the social worker may then draft a policy for the council or modifications to an existing policy for the administration to ratify. There are generally three basic tasks that a family council performs which the social worker needs to consider, and these can be covered in the policy. The basic functions of the council are problem resolution, education, and improving the quality of life for the residents of the facility.

Problem resolution applies to common issues that family members might have, such as missing laundry or complaints related to any of the departments, including medical care, nursing, rehabilitation, recreation, housekeeping, or social services. When an issue is specific to the needs of a particular resident and does not represent a systemic problem, it should not be discussed the public forum of a council meeting, but rather, the social worker should insist that it be addressed in a separate, private meeting.

Education includes helping families understand aspects of how the nursing home functions, the processes of aging, medical diagnoses, insurance information, or anything that relates to the situation of having a loved one who requires nursing home care. While family members of short-term rehabilitation patients are welcome to attend council meetings, in reality, the agendas of the meetings are based primarily on the needs and concerns of family members of permanent residents. Family members can be asked to suggest topics that they might wish to learn about, and the social worker could then engage a speaker from within the facility or from the larger community who is qualified to provide information on the topic at hand. Some topics that I have found to be of interest to family members include Medicare; depression; advance directives such as living wills, healthcare proxies, and powers of attorney; self-care for stress; and tips for a successful visit, to name a few. Tips for a successful visit, for example, is a topic that the social worker, in collaboration with the activities director or facility-contracted mental health professional, can conduct herself, if she wishes.

Finally, the family council's efforts at improving the quality of life for residents of the facility can include any projects that the council wishes to undertake (within the parameters of their role, of course), including bake sales or other projects to raise money for the activities department or sponsoring a holiday party for the residents, for example.

Once the social worker has enlisted the good will and, more importantly, the cooperation of management, her next task is to begin to engage families and invite them to a family council planning meeting. To do this, it is a good idea to contact personally individuals with whom you already have a good relationship and who are likely to participate. In addition, it is wise to personally invite family members who visit frequently and/or who are already involved in the life of the facility. If you have worked with an angry family member who might be known to the administration for being difficult and critical and have helped the family member feel that his or her concerns have been understood, inviting that person to join a family council can result in successfully engaging the family member's energies in a constructive manner.

After approaching some families personally, the social worker can then expand her efforts to publicize a family council planning meeting by mailing invitations to all family members and by posting signs throughout the building.

At the first meeting, it may be advisable to have the administrator, the director of nursing, and key department heads present, in keeping with the effective soldiers' home model of high administrative involvement. This meeting is a time to reaffirm the importance of the family council and to establish a level of trust between family members and the administration. At this time, the functions of the council should be discussed, and the administrator should assure family members that the facility will respond to their concerns and suggestions. At the soldiers' home, the facility's response is recorded in the minutes of that meeting, or, if more time is needed to look into a problem, it is noted in the report of the following meeting. The social worker is a natural choice to be the liaison between the council and the administration and should help the family council president, once officers are elected, to present the families' concerns and make sure they are followed up.

The administration may continue to be involved for one or two subsequent planning meetings—meetings at which members make decisions about the frequency of meetings, meeting time and place, the election and role of officers, arrangements for having minutes typed and mailed, and other important nuts-and-bolts matters. I would recommend that the social worker continue to attend the meetings for a while longer, assisting the council in coming up with a format with which they feel comfortable and in writing a charter document, if desired, as well as coaching the group leader(s) in group facilitation techniques such as checking in with quieter members and tactfully setting limits on those who tend to monopolize the meeting. The social worker can also model leadership roles by focusing on all three aspects of council activity, rather than just problem resolution, maintaining a positive problem-solving approach, and encouraging group members to support one another. Ultimately, the social worker's goal is to have the council function autonomously, with her presence needed only at the beginning and near the end of each session, at the beginning to introduce any new developments in the facility and at the end to elicit a list of concerns to be addressed. But until the council feels ready to take over, the social worker should be prepared to continue to help facilitate the meetings.

As the social worker works with the council toward the goal of empowering them to be autonomous, yet closely connected with the facility, it is important for her, as facility liaison, to develop and to maintain a trusting relationship with the council members and a close working relationship with the council president(s). She should also remain available to the council, and in particular to the president or copresidents and other elected officers, for consultation about group dynamics, council functioning, and assistance with wording of the content of the minutes, if desired. In her successful council, the director at the soldiers' home strongly encouraged council members to resolve any interpersonal difficulties without her intervention if at all possible. She would listen if family members sought her out to "vent" about each other, but in the end, she tried to encourage the individual involved to work things out directly with the other party. This independence from excessive reliance on the staff of the facility on the part of the council is essential, because a council that is overly dependent lacks the ability to give families an effective voice in advocating for their loved ones, who are often unable to express their own needs.

OTHER PROGRAMS FOR FAMILIES

While the family council is the primary vehicle for family involvement in the functioning of the nursing home, the social worker can also encourage family involvement in the community of the nursing home in a number of ways. These include the development of support groups, such as a dementia support group for family members of residents with this condition, as well as working with nurse unit managers and the activities department to promote having simple holiday parties and other special celebrations on each unit to which family members are invited.

Family Support Groups

Often, families shy away from participation in a support group, perhaps because of the stigma of appearing weak and in need of support. Over time, the family council may develop the characteristics of a support group as members get to know and learn to trust one another. However, I have found that there is often need for specialized support groups, which provide education and support about disease such as Alzheimer's, Parkinson's, and multivascular and other dementias. These diagnoses do not affect all of the residents, but they do affect the entire family system of those individuals who suffer them. Leadership training is available for some support groups, for example, from the Alzheimer's Association.[2] An initial focus on an educational component, including guest speakers from the facility and the larger community, is helpful in decreasing any stigma associated with a need for support, thus paving the way for family members to become comfortable attending meetings in which they gradually are able to take advantage of the supportive relationships that develop among group members in this type of setting.

Family Parties on the Units

A simple way to accentuate the feeling of community on a particular unit is to hold a small family/resident/staff gathering on that unit. Holidays and seasonal celebrations are perfect excuses for a party. To facilitate this happening, the social worker can work with the nurse manager to set a date at least a month ahead of time, secure administrative permission, if required, and notify the activities director, who can assist with working with the kitchen to obtain refreshments and perhaps provide live entertainment. Alternatively, music from compact discs or tapes can be used. Add a few decorations, and voilà, a happy occasion is created that brings staff, residents, and family members together for purposes other than care-plan meetings or other professional business. Parties such as these take relatively little time to organize and plan, yet go a long way toward creating positive memories associated with the nursing home. These memories can be preserved and validated by taking pictures of the event to be displayed on the unit and given to loved ones as keepsakes. One way to incorporate this intervention into your practice is to focus on one unit for a particular quarter and to encourage the nursing staff on the unit to take increasing responsibility for initiating and planning the programs in collaboration with the activities department.

Family members are stuck between a rock and a hard place when they make the decision to place a loved one. This act is almost never done by choice but because circumstances make it necessary. Social workers can and should assist families in coping with the stress of this major life transition, most crucially at the time of the initial placement, but also by instituting family councils. In for-profit settings, where family empowerment appears anathema to the agenda of the facility, social workers need to work closely with the administration to negotiate common goals that will lead to the facility's acceptance and support of a strong and effective family council that, at the end of the day, will benefit everybody, as well as of other programs to shore up and strengthen family coping. All this affects the quality of life for the residents with whom the family members are inextricably linked and, in the long run, serves the interests of the facility as client.

Notes

1. The National Citizens' Coalition for Nursing Home Reform, 1828 L Street NW, Suite 801, Washington, D.C. 20036; phone, (202) 332-2276; www.nccnhr.org. The NCCNHR has a Web page devoted to the formation of family councils. This information was developed as part of a project funded by the Maryland Department of Health and Mental Hygiene, Office of Health Care Quality, a five-year project to develop and strengthen family councils in Maryland, and is geared to an audience of family members seeking to initiate their own councils. However, the site contains a wealth of information that can be helpful to social workers seeking to assist families with this initiative. For example, there are tips on setting up bulletin boards in the facility and involving the local ombudsman, along with links to many relevant resources. This Web site also has a listing of local citizens' groups in many states that can serve as valuable resources.

2. The Alzheimer's Association National Office, 225 North Michigan Avenue, Floor 17, Chicago, IL 60601. The Alzheimer's Association is a not-for-profit 50(c)(3) organization. Their Web site is www.alz.org, which has links to local organizations. Their 24/7 Helpline is (800) 272-3900.

Chapter 8

Creating and Sustaining Community in the Nursing Home

IN PREVIOUS CHAPTERS, WE HAVE DISCUSSED PROGRAMS THAT FOCUSED primarily on the needs of residents, staff members, or families. In this chapter, we will consider involving all of these components at once through programs that work synergistically to address the needs of the nursing home as a community, for when they are part of a community, residents can begin to heal the psychic injuries that were created when they were separated from their families and neighborhoods.

To this end, I will describe several programs aimed at enhancing residents' quality of life by creating community through the development of meaningful interactions supported by the use of rituals and ceremonies that validate positive roles for the residents, as well as for staff members and families. The programs that we will discuss include rituals related to death and bereavement such as a memorial tea service, an annual memorial service, and a remembrance table, as well as a program that I developed that helps to create community by creating and validating individual one-to-one relationships between staff members and residents—a program called Caring Hearts at Work. While these programs are presented in their entirety, I encourage the reader to adapt any applicable parts of them to their own unique settings, in order to enhance relationships and build community appropriate to the needs and concerns of your practice.

In many ways, it is rituals and ritualized activities with symbolic value that help to define our public roles in society and thus solidify our experience of individual selfhood. As Patricia and Douglas Suggs (2003) note, " rituals give us a foundation, a sense of stability that we need as we tackle challenges and opportunities that confront us on a daily basis" (pp. 17–18). For that reason, I decided to focus on the purposeful use of various interventions to enhance the existence of positive communal feeling for all those involved in the nursing home setting, particularly the residents. In doing so, I have borrowed from anthropological theory, but also from our own social work heritage. This chapter includes the processes by which I developed programs based on the use of practices, rituals, and cere-monies designed to define roles for the residents in the ambiguous setting of the long-term care institution. It is my hope that the bricolage (Lévi-Strauss, 1966), or "cobbling together" of these various elements and practices will inspire other social workers: combine the fragments of a community culture that exist in your environment, your imagination, and the basic social work skills of relationship development, including positive reframing, problem resolution, and the use of ecological perspective in whatever proportion fits the needs of your resident clients, the facility as client, and your own proclivities. Create a living situation that the residents and caregivers alike can experience as meaningful.

THE NURSING HOME EXPERIENCE: AN ANTHROPOLOGICAL PERSPECTIVE

In 1908, Arnold van Gennep (1960) put forth the concept that some rituals, specifically rites of passage accompanying major life-stage transitions, consist of three phases: preliminal rites (rites of separation), liminal rites (rites of transi-tion), and postliminal rites (rites of incorporation). In her ethnography of the cul-ture in an American nursing home, anthropologist Renée Shield (1988), applying this theory to the context of nursing home placement, noted that the elderly res-idents had undergone a separation from the larger community following a change in status in which they were no longer considered to be fully functional adults. In this ambivalent ("liminal") state, largely avoided by the public, they awaited the final transition that is death without the traditional bonds of friendship and com-monality (*communitas*) among themselves to ease the isolation of their social position.

In the twenty-first century, this situation continues. The initial process by which a resident is admitted to a nursing home sets the tone for the resident's future experience of loneliness in a crowd. In short order, the new admission is whisked into a bed, where, behind closed curtains, he or she receives a thorough medical evaluation. Without intending to, here at the very beginning, the staff in effect performs a ritual that strips away the residents' former identity and places the individual in a dependent role in a way that unfortunately still begs for com-parison to the stigmatization endured by mental patients in the institutions described by Erving Goffman (1961) over forty years ago.

Without robust social work intervention, this course of depersonalization inexorably proceeds as the resident "adjusts" to his or her new living situation. Although our role is not widely understood or acknowledged (neither Shields nor other nursing home ethnographers make explicit mention of the social worker's role in helping to preserve the residents' identities), we as social workers are responsible for balancing the process of medicalization of our clients with our unique perspective of the person-in-situation that will enable the facility to consider each resident's individuality when planning for his or her care. Furthermore, as Elaine Brody (1974) hinted at in her early and comprehensive effort to clarify and define the role of social worker in the nursing home, we can have and should have a significant role to play in modifying the institutional milieux of our settings.

In fact, we have great potential power to help preserve our residents' identities by making changes to established nursing home traditions, which often ignore the individuality of the patients. We can do this, for example, by insisting that the residents' life histories be known and recognized; by specifically and consistantly reporting the residents' former occupations, achievements, and interests to the care-planning team and the caretaking staff; by helping the team to develop personalized care plans based on this information, encouraging family members to bring in (labeled) pictures from the residents' pasts to put on their bulletin boards and keep in albums at their bedsides to share with staff; by encouraging staff to refer to these resources; and by working with our activities directors to develop creative ways of enabling residents to engage in meaningful activities related to the residents' past interests.

Indeed, the development of programs is a way that we can create new rituals and traditions that enhance community in the nursing home and confer the experience of *communitas* among its members. For instance, lingering over breakfast and reading the paper can be a ritualized activity, one that we associate particularly with retired persons and informal socialization with one's peers at the local coffee shop. Based on this cultural concept, a staff member at a nursing home where I worked developed a "Breakfast Club," where residents who were able to participate came to the dining room for the morning meal (a meal generally served bedside in most facilities) in their pajamas and bathrobes, chose from a selection of breakfast foods, and stayed as long as they wished, reading the paper and chatting with their tablemates. The program was enormously successful and resulted in the residents developing new friendships, as well as a renewed sense of purpose in their physical therapy and daily self-care. This small example demonstrates the power of reinacting symbolic associations, in this case related to both social status ("retired persons") and kinship (eating a meal together in one's pajamas), for creating bonds of commonality and reinforcing a sense of personhood. As social workers, we can and should develop and support the use of both secular ceremonies and sacred rituals that provide comfort and security to the residents.

The use of rituals is not an entirely new idea. They have been used in the past by mental health professionals in the context of family systems therapy. Onno van der Hart (1983) used rituals in his practice to help individuals and families heal from illness, cope with transitions in the life cycle, and strengthen family bonds. Moreover, although it was not articulated as such, the use of ritual has had a place in the social work settlement house and community center traditions. Jane Addams and her colleagues encouraged new immigrants to celebrate their cultures of origin through traditional dance, music, and song while adapting to the exigencies of their new country. It is time that we revisit the use of rituals to effect positive systemic changes on behalf of our clients.

As the growing hospice movement recognizes, life exists right up until it ends. Hospice philosophy emphasizes the importance of meeting the physical, emotional, and spiritual needs of the dying, of allowing them to participate actively in their own care, and of respecting their wishes (Andreae, 2000). Our residents may not be actively dying, but they, too, need to have their emotional and spiritual needs met. Of importance to their well-being is a recognition of their personal and social identities. Our elderly residents, in particular, have had many life roles. They generally have cultural similarities related to the larger community from which they come and/or the particular population served by the nursing home. Let us use our social work skills to discover the residents' common and unique roles and then educate our colleagues to join us in recognizing and to celebrating them. In our professional capacity, we can work toward modifying the nursing home environment to that of a community devoted to the reverence not just of life, but of the unique particulars of the life that exists inside its walls. We can help to ensure that the residents' remaining time will be truly imbued with a richness of meaningful relationships and of cultural, spiritual, and personal experiences.

It should be noted, by the way, that not all nursing home residents are elderly. Currently, a trend exists in which younger mentally and physically disabled individuals whose needs cannot be met elsewhere are being housed, often inappropriately, in nursing homes, even though their problems and concerns differ from and may even be at odds with those of the frail elderly who make up the larger part of the nursing home population (Wunderlich & Kohler, 2001). Nursing homes tend to accept such admissions in greater numbers when economic necessity dictates that they do so, and when such clients are admitted, it is sometimes with adverse effects on the safety of all concerned. The task of social workers in such cases is, more often than not, to try to locate a better setting for these clients. But when this is not possible, assuming that these younger individuals can be managed in the nursing home, the developmental needs of this younger population might also be served with programs and perhaps rituals designed to address their life-stage issues.

CELEBRATING LIFE: THE MEMORIAL TEA SERVICE

The memorial tea service is a program that was developed to mark the final rite of passage that is death and to facilitate communal bereavement and the experience of *communitas* among the survivors. In one of the nursing homes where I worked, as often happens, there were no clergy associated with the facility. When someone died, services were held in the deceased's home community by the family, but no particular attention was paid to the grief of the former resident's roommates or peers who were left behind or, for that matter, to the spiritual needs of the staff. Instead, the beds were summarily filled with new paying customers. All of this suppressed acknowledgment of death led to a vague feeling of tension and malaise that affected the morale of all concerned.

In order to begin to remedy this feeling of alienation, I undertook the challenge of finding a forum for the residents, family, and staff members to come together to commemorate the deceased, as well as to reaffirm the importance of the individual to the community. With guidance from a behavioral psychologist with experience in program development (David Danforth, personal communication, 1997), each time someone died at that nursing home, I sought to establish a protocol that provided a structure for people to process their grief that was flexible enough to allow all those who wished to do so to participate to the extent that they felt comfortable. Thus, the memorial tea service began.

The format of this informal service was simple. After obtaining the administrator's permission, I proceeded with a plan to engage the community each month in recognizing and celebrating the lives of those who had passed away during the past four weeks. I notified the families of the deceased and engaged the activities department in helping to spread the word to the residents and staff. I designed the service itself to have a "drop-in" format, which permitted individuals to feel welcome to come in and pay their respects for a few moments or to stay for the duration of the event.

Prior to the service, I obtained pictures of the deceased and prepared statements about them culled from my psychosocial assessments and my knowledge of their personalities. I also selected a song or hymn appropriate to the deceased resident's religious beliefs (for example, "Amazing Grace" or the Twenty-Third Psalm) to be played on a tape or compact disc or sung by a willing staff member with musical ability. Those things, along with a selection of teas and cookies, completed the preparations.

At the time of the event, I made a particular effort to encourage the deceased resident's special friends and roommates to attend, as well as the nurses and certified nurse assistants (CNAs) who had cared for them. In practice, I found that those friends and roommates who had been invited usually welcomed the opportunity to attend. The CNAs also responded well to the opportunity to participate, even if their schedules permitted only a brief appearance, while nurses rarely attended. Administrators verbally expressed their support for the program, but were generally too busy to find the time to drop in. In subsequent planning for similar programs, I learned to engage representatives from these groups more directly in the planning for the services so that they would have a greater investment in the outcome and be more likely be involved in the proceedings.

The service itself began in a low-key manner. While serving tea and cookies, my co-leaders and I tried to guide casual conversation gently to the topic of reminiscence about the deceased. From there, we segued into a recitation of the resident's life stories, encouraging family members to contribute their superior knowledge of the lives of the deceased. From there, we encouraged family, residents, and staff members to share their recollections of the residents as mother, father, sister, brother, friend, or care recipient in the nursing home. The contributions by staff members, who provided evidence of the resident's enduring qualities, for example, of generosity and kindness expressed as "he always saved me his banana from breakfast," were enormously comforting to families and also important to staff members, who might otherwise not have had the opportunity to share the significance of their relationship with the resident with others.

We both permitted and encouraged digressions from the topic at hand, especially when the group found the sadness difficult to bear, but we always came back to the theme of the celebration of the life of each individual. The sessions officially ended with the songs or poems that had been previously selected, but we did not rush the participants to leave because a calm and peaceful feeling was what I desired to prevail. Although many nurses resisted direct participation, family members often made a point of visiting them on the residents' units, providing them an opportunity to say their good-byes.

The elderly residents participated in the services with the poise and grace of those who have witnessed many deaths, and afterward they expressed positive feelings about both the event and the deceased ("He was a good worker, a smart man. . . ."). Their participation in this informal ritual signified to me that they were getting the message that each member of the community was valued and that they, too, would be remembered when their time came.

I noticed a momentary lull in the tense atmosphere after the services. Those of us who had participated in some way shared a brief moment of connection and transcendence that brought us closer together and that felt sustaining. It was a time to catch our breath and ready ourselves for the new arrival.

At a later date, in a different nursing home, I changed the format of this program by incorporating the suggestions of a nurse familiar with the hospice traditions. This innovation involved obtaining real or artificial flowers prior to the service and passing them out to family members, friends, and caregivers of the deceased shortly after most people had settled into the room. Those holding the flowers, which symbolized the spirit of the deceased in the room, were then invited to place them in a vase, where they would remain for the duration of the service and for a few days afterward, a transitional object to ease the abruptness of the loss of that individual. After trying out this practice, I found that a nice way to end the service was to give some of the flowers, particularly if they were real, to family members to take with them, a final gift from those who cared about their loved one. These symbolic gestures were helpful because they engaged residents, family, and staff members in a meaningful ritual signifying both letting go of the deceased and holding on to their memories.

REMEMBRANCE TABLES

Along the lines of using rituals and ceremonies to address the needs of the nursing home community following a death, at the Soldiers' Home, I worked with

Figure 6. Remembrance table for a veteran.

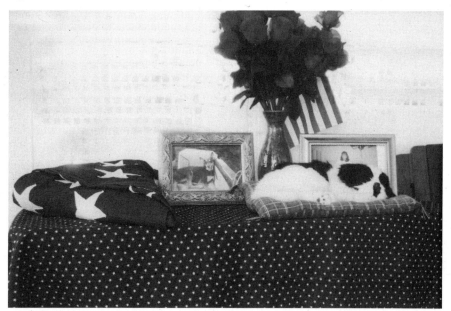

our hospice team and a committee of interested staff members to develop a procedure for helping the community of each barracks-type ward to mourn the loss of a beloved veteran. In that particular setting, the residents would become very close. Sharing the intimate details of each other's lives, the men competed for the nurses' attention, engaged in petty squabbles, and frequently watched out for their peers like brothers. On more than a few occasions, I observed such tenderness as a mute and angry stroke victim holding the hand of a dying neighbor.

When a resident dies on the ward, the death is felt by all the other residents more intensely than if they were not all sharing a room. While this is a positive sign of the existence of community, it also places the residents at risk for feelings of loss and depression, particularly if the bed is summarily filled by a new occupant. In fact, our remembrance tradition began when one of the nurses remarked, following a difficult year when many residents died, that at least in the past, the bed had sat empty for a number of weeks, allowing the veterans and workers to adjust to the absence of the deceased as they contemplated the vacant space. In the current economic climate, no such luxury exists. The effects of unacknowledged, unaddressed grief were palpable. As I noted in chapter 3, the residents bitterly verbalized their own fears of being next, withdrew into depression, and/or acted out their feelings with belligerent behaviors.

In fact, it was the very clear evidence of the veterans' grief for their fallen comrades, that fateful year on 2 North, that brought nurse manager Linda and me to the realization that something needed to be done, and that set in motion the process by which our two-part bereavement protocol was created, including both the remembrance tables described in this section and the annual memorial service for the whole nursing home discussed in the next section.

Initially, unsure of how to proceed with the upset residents of 2 North, Linda and I called a meeting with the bereavement coordinator of our contracted hospice service, with whom we had worked extensively in the past when a newly admitted resident on that ward—a person with AIDS and opportunistic lung cancer who was estranged from his family and who insisted on dying alone, which he proceeded to do in his own way, pulling the covers over his head at all times except for those moments when he managed to get himself out of bed to wheel himself in his wheelchair (oxygen and all) out to smoke a cigarette. While my training indicated that this was his right, it was at least as hard on me, the unit social worker, as on the nursing staff that he refused even to consider hospice services. The hospice worker helped us, as a team, to come to terms with our collective sense of helplessness in this situation, holding meetings in which, as a team, we were able to express our feelings and ultimately to feel empowered in allowing him to determine the manner of his own death.

However, after his and many more difficult deaths, the residents were expressing feelings of hopelessness and helplessness, as well as neediness and excessive aggression (I recall one gentleman flinging the walker of the newly admitted patient in the recently vacated bed next to him because it was inappropriately parked in his area). We again called in our hospice consultant. With her assistance, the nurse manager and I began to conceive of ways in which we could enable the struggling ward to come together, not only to grieve their losses but to reassure the surviving residents that they, too, would be remembered when their time came.

One of our interventions, the remembrance table protocol, involved setting up a small display on the unit. I initially thought of this as an altar, but the rest of the staff was averse to this designation, with its religious connotation, and the intensity of their objection to this term almost derailed the whole project before it even got off the ground, a lesson in being sensitive to the culture of the facility, as well as in having the staff members share in the development of a project from its inception in order to feel comfortable with the result. The remembrance table, as I came to call it, held such items as a picture of the deceased veteran, an American flag, flowers, and personal mementoes, such as a cap inscribed with his branch of military service. The table was to be set up, at the discretion of the unit manager and unit social worker, a few days after a death and to be left in place for about a week. Initially, we envisioned a small service associated with the assembly of the table, but in practice, this procedure became unwieldy, and simply setting up the table while engaging the comments of whoever happened to be nearby proved to be sufficient for our purposes.

Acceptance for this procedure involved not only our presenting the concept to our peers at a morning staff meeting (where it was initially met with resistance, due to the language that I used to describe it) but having a meeting with our hospice team and administration, where a formal document describing our bereavement protocol was presented and approved, along with permission to form a bereavement committee to assist us in implementing our program.

The remembrance table is now accepted as one of the usual routines at the facility. If I do not set it up on a timely basis, the staff reminds me to do so. It is clearly beneficial to staff members, who think that the tables are beautiful and sometimes add their own touches to the arrangements. They bring the families to see them, thus validating to both the families and to themselves that the resident was indeed valued in what was in fact a small community.

Since this is a how-to book, a word of advice is indicated here. It is a good idea to gather photographs and mementos to be used for the table before the body is removed to the funeral home, otherwise, it is more difficult to find a decent picture of the deceased and other objects for the table. It is, of course, necessary to obtain the family's permission to use their loved one's personal belongings for this purpose. This actually offers a wonderful opportunity to let family members know about the table and about the importance that the facility places on personally remembering their loved one. If photographs of the deceased are not available, these may sometimes be found in the residents' identifying information in their records, either in their charts or stored on the facility's computer system.

There are situations where setting up a remembrance table is inadvisable, and this is something that must be decided between the social worker and the unit manager on each unit. Most notably, this intervention is not especially appropriate for a dementia unit, where the residents might become confused or upset by the display (and would probably dismantle it in short order). The bereavement committee remains available to discuss ongoing modifications to the program, such as a recent idea to build shelves on each unit designated for use as remembrance places, a concept that not only speaks to efficiency but to the incorporation of this life-affirming social ritual into the medicalized environment.

ANNUAL MEMORIAL SERVICES

An annual memorial service is an adjunct to the remembrance table program that provides an opportunity for the entire nursing home to express its unity in honoring the dead, and in doing so, it also validates the importance of the living residents in the community. Moreover, the memorial service addresses the needs of families in a more direct and formal way than the remembrance tables on the units.

At the Soldiers' Home, the bereavement committee met several times, both formally and informally, over the course of a few months, planning the program for our first annual memorial service, starting with a general outline and working out all of the specifics, down to the smallest details of procuring adequate space, ordering food, making sure microphones and our accordion were in working order, and so on. Our hospice consultant provided us with a sample program for our first annual event, and we used this as a guideline in creating our own. The theme our service was "The Importance of Remembering." Since we wished to make the service inclusive and ecumenical, we requested that Catholic, Protestant, and Jewish clergy or leaders in their faith communities prepare a short talk on this subject as it relates to their religion. In addition, some committee members volunteered to conduct readings or to read poems related to the program's theme, while others identified individuals who might be counted on to present such material. A nurse, a certified nursing assistant (CNA), and I all agreed to give a speech on the importance of remembering as it relates to our jobs, and we recruited a family member to discuss this subject from her point of view. Since the facility is a military one, we were fortunate to have the services of an honor guard. Finally, a contact with someone affiliated with a wonderful Baptist choir provided us with music for our program.

Once we decided on the specifics of the affair, we proceeded to publicize the event. We made posters, placed a notice in the facility newsletter, and asked the family council to spread the word about this occasion. We also created invitations which we sent to all the family members of residents who had died within the preceding year. In order to personalize the event even further, we specified in the invitations that family members who wished to do so might bring a photograph of their loved one for display on a remembrance wall. While we had initially conceptualized this as a large piece of paper mounted on an actual wall, in its final form it consisted of two suitably decorated poster boards mounted for display on standing easels in the front of our auditorium, with a table between them holding still more photographs. This served as a focal point where service participants gathered and shared their feelings as they looked at the pictures together.

The service itself was astonishingly beautiful, the whole ending up being so much more cohesive and meaningful than the sum of its parts. It was not without its glitches, such as when a dormitory resident valiantly representing the Jewish community at the home developed a severe case of stage fright, but moments such as these served to make the production even more human and poignant. It was truly a time when the community felt united, a ceremony that helped us not only to honor our dead, but to celebrate our identity as a veterans' organization. As soon as the service was over, people began to plan improvements for the next year's ceremony.

The Soldiers' Home has a unique identity, and not all facilities would have the occasion to use such a patriotic theme for either a remembrance table program or an annual memorial service. Memorial observances in other nursing homes would have their own unique features based on commonalities (and differences) among their resident population. For instance, many homes are local, and the service might celebrate the residents' contributions to the greater community during their lifetimes. In any case, while the topic sounds fairly grim, memorial programs are actually uplifting rituals by which social workers can help define and validate the importance of individual lives and strengthen the bonds of communal identity.

THE CARING HEARTS PROGRAM

There are other rituals and ceremonies that can help to enrich the experience of living in a nursing home. One such program that I helped to create was called Caring Hearts at Work. This endeavor brought together residents, staff members, the administration, and families in the formation of caring individual

Figure 7. Caring Hearts employee-resident match pose for a picture.

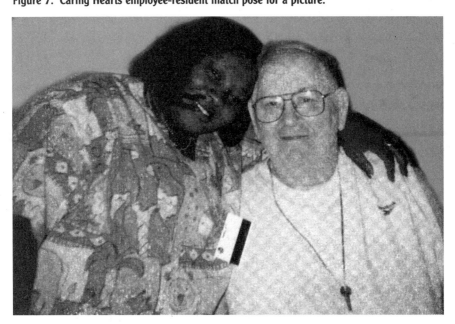

relationships between residents and staff members. To that end, I collaborated
with my coworkers to match interested staff members with residents to spend
some quality time together. Participants were allowed to spend at least twenty
minutes of their work time socializing with their match. The concept for match-
ing residents with staff members was one that I borrowed from a colleague, Joe
Pelland, who presented the idea at a nursing home social work conference. The
title of the program and the form that it ultimately took were my own and my
colleagues' contributions.

As in my work in the area of bereavement, I was careful to involve other key
members of the staff in this program. I initially presented the concept for this
endeavor to my peers as a project for the behavioral committee, which I chaired
as the facility social worker. Our mission was to address concerns about the residents' moods as well as any disruptive behaviors they may have exhibited, prefer-
ably doing so without the use of psychotropic medication. Since positive behavioral modification techniques were the committee's intervention of choice,
according to its mission, I felt that this forum was an appropriate place to launch
this experiment. I hoped the result would be decreased depression and a lessen-
ing of the need to act out on the part of the residents as their emotional needs
were being met through their special relationship with a staff member.

After gaining the approval of the committee, which included the activities director, an occupational therapist, and a nurse, I wrote up a proposal for the administrator which was reviewed by my collaborators. After some discussion, we made some revisions to the document and submitted it to the administrator for approval, and it was accepted.

We recruited interested staff members and allowed them to chose a resident to be their Caring Hearts partner. About twelve employees initially signed up. We gave those workers a heart sticker to wear on their badges, signifying their status as members of this program. According to our rules, which we explained to them verbally and in writing, they were allowed to visit with their resident anywhere in the facility or on the grounds for a total of twenty minutes per week, with the consent of their supervisor, and to spend additional time with their match, if desired. We clarified that we expected the relationship to be a caring and professional one and discouraged staff members from sharing overly intimate details of their own personal lives, focusing instead on getting to know the resident better, learning their life stories, and discovering commonalities as well as differences between the lives of their residents and themselves. A requirement was that employees submit a brief check-off form indicating the residents' mood and concerns, as well as a comment about the week's visit(s). This allowed me, as the social worker, to monitor the program's effectiveness and the residents' concerns in general.

Figure 8. Caring Hearts duo spending time together.

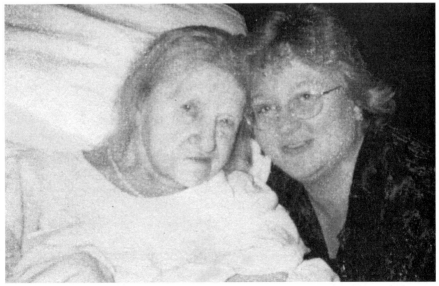

As an incentive for employees to participate in the Caring Hearts Program, the administration agreed to provide a monthly luncheon for staff participants. At these luncheons, the activities director and I facilitated a discussion of each employee's experiences, validated their achievements in developing trusting relationships, and helped the group solve problems involving any concerns that the workers might have. In this way, we modeled caring, constructive interactions for the staff. We also provided education about the importance of reminiscence and taught the staff members some basic life-review techniques, such as asking questions about pictures in a resident's room, about his or her occupation, hobbies, family, past holiday celebrations, and seasonal activities, as appropriate.

Eventually, the program grew to include almost forty staff member/resident pairs. Some of the relationships that developed were extraordinary. Several employees visited their Caring Hearts partners on weekends, bringing their children or pets to show the residents. Strikingly, a very demented resident recognized her staff member by name, even though the patient had not made any other intelligible verbalizations for years. Moreover, staff members began to advocate actively for their charges. A physical therapist, for example, made sure her Caring Heart partner was walked daily, something that had not occurred prior to her intervention. Finally, in care-plan meetings, families often mentioned their appreciation for the Caring Heart staff member assigned to their loved one and noted that the residents looked forward to these special visits.

In order to continue to flourish, the Caring Hearts Program, like a garden, needed to be constantly cultivated and tended. I kept the program growing by recognizing the efforts of Caring Hearts staff members and the relationships that resulted from their work with the residents. I wrote an article about the program that was published in the local newspaper. I also took pictures of Caring Hearts duos each year, displaying them as a collage in a prominent location. Thus, Caring Hearts participants acquired a certain cachet that encouraged other staff members to join the program. I also held a contest where staff members competed to design a logo. We had the winning entry (two smiling hearts holding hands) made into T-shirts which we sold at cost to employees, who in turn were permitted to wear them as part of the dress code. The T-shirts were in great demand, and cheerful red hearts appeared daily among the white and pastel floral uniforms. In visible ways, the rituals associated with the Caring Hearts Program helped to humanize the medicalized culture of the facility.

One effect of the Caring Hearts Program that was not so positive, however, was that, having developed meaningful bonds with the elderly residents, staff members were now more vulnerable to the loss of those relationships due to death. In a staff luncheon, one worker reported that when her match died, she cried all the way home. We talked about how hard it is to lose someone that you care about. This occurrence brought me back full circle to the issue of bereavement, because life is inevitably, inextricably entwined with death, especially when working with those in the late stages of their development. I instituted the monthly memorial tea services in this nursing home, which I had not previously done, and Caring Hearts staff members quite often attended, even in their off hours.

From my experience in creating these programs, I would recommend being somewhat rigorous in developing procedures to measure and quantify the outcomes of one's interventions. In the case of the Caring Hearts Program, it would be possible to compare depression scores on such instruments as the Folstein Mini-Mental Status Examination or the Cornell Scale for Depression in Dementia pre-match, at three-month, six-month, and yearly intervals. Behavioral changes could be compared on the Multiple Data Set administered in every facility. The behavior check-off sheets filled out by Caring Hearts Program participants could also be tracked over time. The information obtained through these methods could be helpful to a facility in its marketing services, which would in turn increase the value of the program to the administration and ensure continued administrative support for a this type of project. In terms of the remembrance tables, resident moods and behavior could be similarly tracked through the administration of depression protocols and comparison of MDS dates for the residents before and after the program is instituted on a particular unit. For all programs, documenting staff and family comments can serve as indicators of the success of the endeavor.

Nursing homes, like hospitals and similar institutions, remove the elderly from the mainstream of society in order to care for them, and as has always been the case, this type of care engenders an existential crisis for the residents. No longer valued for their economic contributions and not yet dead, they remain in a marginalized netherworld, dependent on attendants who do not really know them, with no ties to each other and frayed bonds with their family members, who no longer know how to treat them. This situation, while admittedly grim, is an opportunity for nursing home social workers to use their understanding of systems, relationships, and human behavior to develop programs that go a long way toward helping our clients to reestablish meaningful identities.

Chapter 9

The Art of Paperwork

PAPERWORK IS A FACT OF LIFE FOR A SOCIAL WORKER IN A NURSING HOME. Lest the reader misunderstand the importance of timely and accurate paperwork in the overall scheme of things, this chapter focuses on the subject of documentation and suggests a method for managing this important aspect of the nursing home social worker's responsibilities. There are many ways to organize one's paperwork, but the benefit of this particular method is that it involves an effective way to conceptualize clinical information about one's clients.

As I've mentioned before, I have found that the best time to do the assessment of a new resident is immediately after their arrival. This is especially beneficial because it gives the social worker the opportunity to meet with the family, if they are present, and obtain from them psychosocial information that the new resident might not be able to provide due to cognitive limitations. Sometimes the social worker is not notified when a new admission arrives. This can be remedied by working with the admissions director, MDS coordinator, or nurse unit manager to arrange to be informed of new arrivals.

Whatever forms are used by your facility, I have found that there is no substitute for a good old-fashioned narrative (it does not have to be long) reporting the following information (at minimum):

> Name and nickname(s) that the resident prefers to be called
> Marital status (and existence of a significant other, if this is the case)
> Ethnicity (important and often neglected in social service assessments)
> Religion (including comments on formal church/synagogue attendance and/or other spiritual practices)
> Major diagnoses
> Place of birth
> Number of siblings
> Military history
> Occupation
> Children

Hobbies and interests (very important for future care plans)

Basic support network (family members and significant others on whom the person counts for emotional sustenance as well as possible physical assistance)

Comments on the patient's understanding and response to medical condition and placement

Comments on mood and mental status

Finally, a sentence or two about how the social worker plans to address this particular resident's needs based on the above noted information.

Here's an example of how these elements can take on the form of a narrative.

Case study

Mildred Goldstein (who prefers to be called "Millie") is an eighty-four-year-old widowed Jewish woman of Russian descent. She was admitted to Sunny Valley Nursing Home from General Hospital with a diagnosis of right-sided stroke, coronary artery disease, depression, and arthritis.

Millie was born in New York, the oldest of three children. Her siblings have been deceased for more than ten years now. Millie completed high school and married Paul at age twenty. She had five children: John, Stephen, Esther Cohen, Sarah Goldstein, and Bob. All are highly successful in the fields of law, medicine, and business. She worked as an administrative secretary in the clothing industry. Her husband Paul, a tailor, died twenty years ago, and she moved to elderly housing, where she lived until being admitted to this facility. There she had Meals on Wheels from the Elderly Commission and homemaker services to assist with housecleaning, laundry, and transportation to doctors' appointments. She had a cat, Puff, now staying with a friend. She has been estranged from her children for many years, but recently Sarah and Bob, who live locally, have become involved with her care. She expresses positive feelings about their recent visits at the hospital but is concerned about "being a burden," because they "have their own lives and careers." Millie enjoyed playing canasta with a group of friends in her building. She is alert and oriented to person and place and knows the season and the year but not the month. Her mood is irritable and angry at times. She states that she wants to go home but has limited motivation for therapy, according to the hospital reports. She denies any concerns about her physical limitations, including inability to transfer from bed to chair and incontinence of the bladder. The staff express concerns about her ability to return home safely. The social worker is to provide support to the resident around adjustment to losses of health and independence and placement in the facility, encourage her to participate in care and the discharge-planning process with her family and interdisciplinary team, and help her process her feelings about recent stressors and major life changes.

Developing an Initial Care Plan from the Patient's Point of View

This basic information already tends to suggest a care plan by the picture it paints, in broad narrative outlines, of the client and her situation. Medical care plans are usually organized, for better or for worse, into three parts: problem, goal, and approaches. Since we are obligated to take this somewhat negative approach to addressing this woman's situation, we will, of course, do so, but we will also be sure to include her strengths and supports in the care plan, and, above all, we will write it from her point of view.

Her "problem," as she sees it, is that she wants to go home, but is not allowed to, which naturally makes her angry—angry at her body, for refusing to cooperate with her any more, angry at the nursing home, at her caregivers there, and possibly angry at her children, to whom she has feels she dedicated her life in order to make them independent and highly successful, but who now appear too wrapped up in their own families and busy, fast-paced lifestyles to bother with her.

Trying to put ourselves in her shoes, we can sense the client may have some denial about the extent of her medical condition. This is probably necessary for her protection against being overwhelmed by her many losses. She should not, of course, be disabused of her hopes, although the social worker and team should be careful to present the realities of her situation gently. The social worker should monitor her mood and mental status for symptoms of clinical depression, and since she already has this diagnosis (it appears that this condition was diagnosed at the hospital following her stroke), the social worker should advocate for referral to formal psychiatric services at the nursing home to monitor her conditions and psychotropic medication.

One caveat: always write your care plans as if the patient and her family will read them. That way, in care-plan meetings, communication will be more straightforward and forthright. As well, you will not have to worry about potential problematic situations where the family requests to see the chart for one reason or another. Here, for example, is how the narrative of Mrs. Goldstein's basic information can be fit into the Procrustean bed of the care-plan formula.

Case study

Problem: Mrs. Goldstein is coping with adjustment to multiple recent stressors, including health and independence losses related to recent stroke, nursing home placement, and separation from her cat. She very much wants to go home, but staff members have concerns about her ability to do so safely, due to difficulty with transfers and bladder incontinence. Also related to her stroke, Mrs. Goldstein is experiencing symptoms of depression, irritability, and lack of motivation. Mrs. Goldstein is an independent woman who is proud of her achievements in having a career and raising capable, successful children. In the past, she has been reluctant to ask her children for assistance, but since her illness, she has needed to do so, and her children have been available and are openly supportive. Millie has a strong Jewish faith and many friends in her building.

As the reader can see, the social worker has made a point of emphasizing the client's biographical information in an ongoing effort to educate staff members about who this person is and to encourage them to interact with her based on that information. This also prompts us all to follow up on this information in planning for her care. Since we have discovered that she has a strong Jewish faith, we need to consider the possibility that she may require a kosher diet and to check with her to see if this is the case. If it is, we must work with the dietary department to provide this. In her case, it turned out that she did not keep kosher but did not eat shellfish or any pork products. In exploring her religious and spiritual preferences, we should also determine if she would like visits from her local rabbi. If so, the social worker can help to arrange this. As we'll see, all of these interventions will go in the "Approaches" section of the care plan.

In the "Goals" section, we will again consider the situation from the patient's point of view.

Case study

Goals: Mrs. Goldstein will achieve and maintain her maximum level of independent functioning in the least restrictive setting. She will maintain her ties with her family, her community, and her cat to the extent possible. She will participate in the care and discharge planning process as the interdisciplinary care-plan team evaluates her ability to achieve her rehabilitation goals of independent transfers and toileting. Mrs. Goldstein will feel supported by the facility staff. Her spiritual needs will be addressed. She will express her feelings, if she wishes to do so, about her present stressors and the discharge planning process.

In the "Approaches" section, we will try to use as many of the patient's supports and interests as we can to address her needs.

Case study

Approaches: The social worker will meet with Mrs. Goldstein to provide support and to encourage her to attend her care-plan meetings, discuss her medical condition with her doctor, and express her feelings about adjustment to her recent stroke and her progress toward her rehabilitation goal of returning to the community.

The social worker will assist Millie in contacting her local rabbi, because she wishes him to visit.

The dietary department will honor Millie's preference not to eat pork or shellfish. The social worker will provide outreach to family and support to them concerning major life changes in the family's situation due to the patient's illness and to encourage positive visits with the patient as they all adjust to their new family roles.

The social worker will encourage family members to bring in photo albums and will arrange brief visits with grandchildren. The daughter plans to arrange to bring the cat for a visit and has obtained a picture of the cat for the resident to put on her bulletin board, along with several pictures of her family and grandchildren.

The social worker will encourage Millie to maintain contact with her friends through phone calls.

The social worker will introduce the resident to several another women living in the facility who play canasta.

This is a fairly complicated care plan because the patient's situation is complex. This case involves a patient admitted for short-term care who may or may not be able to go home. As you can see, we do not know for certain what the outcome of her rehabilitation treatment will be. Although at this time the patient returning home appears unlikely, she has expressed this wish, and there is no question of her mental competence. Therefore, in addressing the patient's expressed desire, the social worker in this case, together with the patient, her family, and the interdisciplinary team, should consider patient and family resources and assets, public and private homecare agencies, as well as possible assisted living or supportive housing in the community.

Even if Millie is unable to return home, the social worker and team should continue to present information about that goal to her in relationship to her overall rehabilitation goals. This emphasizes the fact that long-term care is not a decision that the facility has made unilaterally but is the current situation based on Millie being at this time unable to meet her rehabilitation goals. One should never take away a patient's hope.

In the meantime, the stage is set for Millie to strengthen her ties with her family, continue to practice her faith, and begin to develop new friendships in the nursing home. All of this falls under the rubric of her care-plan goal of achieving and maintaining her maximum level of independence in the least restrictive setting.

This care plan may have taken some time to develop, but it will also save time, for example, by avoiding negative outcomes such as a premature decision on the part of the facility that the patient cannot return home, a failure to assist the patient in mobilizing her support network and in helping her develop new supports in the facility, as well as something so seemingly minor as a failure to recognize her dietary needs, which could negatively affect her relationship and that of the family with the facility. Writing the care plan from the patient's point of view also helps staff members to empathize with her situation and mitigates against the tendency of staff members to react to a patient's anger by emotional withdrawal, which would also be detrimental to her care.

MAKING A MEMORY CARD

I am indebted to Dr. David Danforth, a behavioral psychologist who invented the "card method" in his own practice and generously shared this deceptively simple and highly efficient and effective technique for conceptualizing and remembering client information.

To use this method, once the care plan is written, the nursing home social worker constructs an index card and tries to commit to memory the basic information about this case as she has developed it from the patient's personal information, as in the example illustrated below.

Case study

Mildred Goldstein ("Millie") Unit 6B

DOB: 5/4/24

Diagnosis: <u>Right-sided stroke</u>, coronary artery disease, depression, arthritis

Medications: Aspirin, <u>Zoloft (50 milligrams per day)</u>.

Social History: 84-year-old widowed Jewish woman of Russian descent, born in Boston, 3 siblings, high-school education, worked as a secretary for a clothing company, 5 children. Had a cat. Liked to attend synagogue, play canasta, read NY Times.

Because the social worker must keep the information about numerous patients in mind at the same time, having a system based on cards in this format provides a structure for her to think about and remember her cases. As I've done in the example, I like to underline information related to psychiatric diagnoses and medical conditions that are known to cause psychiatric symptoms, such as a stroke, multiple sclerosis, Parkinson's disease, Alzheimer's disease, and so on, because this reminds me to be alert for such concerns when dealing with that patient.

WHEN TO WRITE A CARE PLAN

Over the years, I have found that it is better to write too many care plans than too few. Being involved in writing care plans promotes an awareness of a patient's case (for the social worker and others) and involves the social worker in conversations with members of the interdisciplinary team about the patient's concerns, promoting collaborative team efforts on behalf of the patient. Attending a morning meeting or department head meeting is a very good way to be apprised of situations that may require a care plan. Alternatively, if this is not possible, listening to nursing rounds at shift change on a regular basis and/or reading nursing logs on each unit are other ways to obtain this important information about significant changes in the patients' lives and medical conditions.

Some situations that call for a new patient care plan include the following:

◆ Significant medical changes (for example, new g-tube placement, amputation of a limb, a new diagnosis of cancer) that are likely to affect the resident's self-image and sense of well being and to bring up issues of mortality. Positive medical changes are also important to a care plan, such as making significant progress in ambulation or toward another goal. Such changes may potentially lead to the initiation of discharge planning or other social service interventions.

- Cognitive changes, for better or for worse.
- Behavioral changes/emotional changes (it is important to try as a team to determine the precipitant or cause for these in developing a care plan).
- Significant family events (for example, death of a family member, the anniversary of an event of great significance to the resident, or an important wedding that the resident may be planning to attend).

A care plan should also be instituted when a resident is deemed by the doctor to have a terminal condition. An example of an "end of life" care plan for Mr. Jones, who has end-stage Alzheimer's disease, might be as follows.

Case study

Problem: End of life; patient has late-stage Alzheimer's diagnosis with very limited prognosis, per M.D.

Goals: Mr. Jones will feel safe and secure in his environment, as evidenced by family reports and staff observation of the patient's verbalizations and facial expressions. Mr. Jones will be free from pain or discomfort as determined by nursing assessments, staff observations, and family reports. Dignity will be maintained. Spiritual needs will be addressed. Family will feel supported by the staff.

Approaches: Hospice services were initiated by nursing per order of M.D. Nursing is to monitor for pain and make appropriate interventions as indicated in collaboration with hospice and M.D. Because Mr. Jones ("Bill") loved big-band music, his favorite selections will be played on his CD player at bedside daily. Mr. Jones is to be visited by the hospice chaplain and social worker is to contact his parish priest per family request. The social worker and nursing staff are to provide support to family members during their visits, and the social worker is to provide outreach to family as indicated.

OTHER REASONS FOR CARE PLANS

A care plan of some sort is required when a resident has a condition affecting his or her communication, such as a visual or hearing impairment, for example. The social worker should try to ensure that such a care plan is in place and, if it is not, should help to initiate one. If a care plan for legal blindness, aphasia/inability to communicate verbally, or hearing loss, to cite a few examples, is in place, there is almost always an opportunity for the social worker to add a social service goal and/or approach. Note that adding to a care plan written by someone else should always be done with their prior permission, because you expect the same consideration from others.

A care plan is always required when there is a question of the resident being discharged and if the resident requests to be discharged, even if this goal is deemed to be unrealistic.

It is important to have a care plan to address issues of competency that are being confronted but that are not yet resolved, such as when guardianship is pending. Copies of legal papers related to this issue, such as medical certificates (papers completed by a psychiatrist or M.D. addressing their assessment of someone's competency to manage their own affairs) and temporary and permanent guardianship decrees should be kept in a legal section of the resident's chart, along with his or her advance directives, health care proxy, power of attorney, and other similar documents.

PROGRESS NOTES

Social workers are mandated to write quarterly notes on each resident every ninety days. This can be done after care-plan meetings, assuming care-plan meetings adhere to the schedule mandated by nursing home regulations. The benefit of doing this at this time is that the social worker can note resident and family attendance at care-plan meetings in her progress notes. Alternatively, the social worker can develop some sort of progress-note "tickler file" with an index card for each resident, separating the cards by month and indicating when the next note is due. However, if she uses that system, she should also write an additional note stating that a care-plan meeting was held, particularly if staff and/or family members attend these meetings, and state whether or not they are in agreement with the care plan. Parenthetically, because resident advocacy is one of the social worker's jobs, it is important that she be assertive in making sure that the resident is invited to care-plan meetings, negotiating with staff members who may not think this is important, in order to ensure that each resident has this opportunity to have his or her concerns heard and addressed by the interdisciplinary care-plan team.

Realistically, the mere fact that quarterly care-plan meetings are done is a minimum requirement for the social service job, and the fact that they are done sometimes is seen as more important by reviewers than what the notes actually say. Be that as it may, some of the things that a social service note should indicate are: recent hospitalizations, the resident's mood and mental status, any significant incidents, socialization with family and friends, and participation in activities. What follows is an example of a social service progress note.

Case study

Mrs. Smith was hospitalized from December 6 through December 8, 2007, with pneumonia at the General Hospital. She is presently at her baseline, medically. Ada is alert and oriented to self and place but not to time. Except for when she was not feeling well, her mood has been positive this quarter. She enjoys knitting on her own, socializing with peers and staff, and attends church weekly. Her daughter visits several times a month and has taken her on an overnight outing over the Thanksgiving holiday. The social worker is to work with the activities department to encourage Ada and her friends to work together to knit some items for the upcoming holiday bazaar.

The social worker also should document in the chart any phone calls made to family members or collaterals and other case-management assistance that she may have provided. These notes need not be elaborate and should avoid disclosing information that it is not important for other team members to know about the case. In addition, she should note hospitalizations (the date of the resident's admission and return, as well as the reason for the hospitalization) and any significant incidents in the resident's life. If these incidents have an effect on the resident's coping over time, then a new care plan should be written to reflect the resident's changing needs.

Finally, when there has been an instance in which the resident may have experienced a traumatic event, the social worker should follow this situation, make referrals to other services as necessary, and make frequent notes in the care plan as to how the resident is coping with the aftermath of the incident. If this situation was the result of what might be considered abuse, of course, the situation should be investigated and reported according to facility policy and state and federal regulations. While the resident's responses to this type of unfortunate situation are recorded in the chart, the actual details of such an incident are not considered to be a part of the medical record but instead are reported separately on forms designed for internal facility use.

THE ART OF PAPERWORK—AND LIFE

Paperwork is part of the fabric of a social worker's professional life. While the habit of keeping track of our activities for and on behalf of our clients is awkward and cumbersome at first, it eventually becomes second nature. Everybody develops a system that works best for them, and this chapter describes one that the author has adopted. The core concept of this system is to conceptualize each individual resident in terms of their specific personal information and use this information to develop a plan of care that is tailored to that person's needs in their particular situation. The benefit of all this is that you avoid the need to use generic, impersonal care plans, write excessively formulaic progress notes, and engage in other mind-numbing activities that divert our attention from the fact that we are dealing with living human beings.

Chapter 10

Evaluating

IN THIS BOOK, I HAVE ADDRESSED REMINISCENCE-BASED PROGRAMS, ART-based programs, and other programs for nursing home residents, those with and without cognitive losses, and explored some of the reasons, clinical and theoretical, as well as practical and institutional, why such programs are desirable. In previous chapters, I have touched on the value of evaluating these programs, both as ways to aid in their development and in order to provide arguments for their continued evolution and support, and suggested some ad hoc ways to do so. However, it is both possible and desirable to construct a more formal framework for program evaluation.

This chapter will relate in greater depth the process by which an assessment framework might be developed retroactively to evaluate one of my programs, the current events group. The purpose of this exercise is to demonstrate on a practical level how we can begin to incorporate evaluation research into our established clinical practices and to suggest ways in which we can include the use of program evaluation in the development of future programs in order to measure and improve our own effectiveness and raise our standards of accountability.

Ideally, as I've noted, assessment is part of the original planning process for program development. In real life, this does not always happen. The programs discussed in this book were based on the theoretical benefits of approaches such as life review and on my own clinical experience. They did not have the benefit of a formal evaluation process as part of their development. I therefore had to find a way to assess them going forward in order to establish a baseline for assessing my clients' progress over time. For the purpose of this discussion, I have adapted a framework developed as an arts program evaluation guideline to the assessment of this multifunctional group, the current events group mentioned above (Dreeszen, 2003).

EVALUATION PROTOCOL

I) Identify long-term goals of the program, expressed in terms that reflect social work values. In discussing the goal of the program, theory should be considered by conducting a literature review.

II) Specify the indicators of success for the program: evidence that the objective was (or was not) accomplished.

III) Specify data sources: where the evidence will be found.

IV) Clarify evaluation methods, such as who gathers the data, and how the information will be analyzed.

V) Explain how the evaluation results will be used; who will receive the report and for what purpose.

ETHICAL CONSIDERATIONS

In establishing a formal evaluation framework for this program, I had to contend with a number of ethical concerns. One was the mandate that social workers must obtain the informed consent of participants in a study. Since this study met the criteria for a performance evaluation study similar to others that are customarily undertaken by the performance improvement committee for internal use at the agency, it turned out that no special permission other than the patients' verbal consent was needed.

Another ethical issue is the necessity of adhering to agency policies and procedures (see Brun, 2005). Here, I ensured that the study did so by discussing it with social services and nursing administrators, as well as with key staff members involved with the study, including nurse managers, the activities director, and other social workers.

An additional ethical issue involved use of the results of this study. In this case, the results would be limited to internal agency use for the purpose of program assessment and planning.

A final ethical issue that was of concern to me as a social worker was the dilemma of possibly needing to exclude patients from participating in order to establish a control group. This concern led to our collective agency decision to incorporate into the study all of the new residents who would be able to qualify for participation in it. In this way, the relationship between participation in the group and positive well-being could still be studied, although the study would be less rigorously scientific than if a control group were established. It appears from the literature of social service evaluation that this type of compromise in the interest of meeting the needs of clients is acceptable and appropriate.

As circumstances would have it, administrative and plant changes in the facility dictated that a cohort of about thirty-five long-term care residents from another building would be moving into a new unit in the wing where the group was held. I decided to evaluate all of the residents in the new group who might be eligible to participate in the current events program and to compare the physical and emotional functioning of residents who did and did not take part in this group. The results would not constitute a research study with internal and external validity, but it would be suggestive of the relationships between my goals, their implementation, and a result. The results would have heuristic value. What follows is a completed evaluation guideline for the program under consideration.

I. GOALS OF THE PROGRAM

Many goals of the current events group extended beyond the scope of discussing the daily news. They were: to enhance the residents' sense of individual identity, to foster community, and thus to help the residents improve and maintain an optimal level of emotional, social, cognitive, and physical functioning.

The Background and Values of the Residents

This program targeted residents with cognitive skills ranging from intact cognition to moderate dementia who were able to process information and who had fairly good long-term memory. The veterans in the nursing home at the soldiers' home are almost all male, mostly of Irish or Italian descent, reflecting the population of the surrounding community, although some had other ethnic backgrounds, such as German, Polish, or French Canadian. About three-quarters of the residents fought in World War II, and almost a quarter were Korean War vets. A few are Vietnam veterans.

In general, about half of the residents had a high-school education and half did not, having been raised at a time when they had to go to work and support their families. Many were self-educated, particularly about history and current events. Most took an interest in movies, sports, and science. Most had been married, and a significant number of the residents had experienced estrangement from their families due to a past history of alcohol abuse, possibly related to an attempt to self-medicate symptoms of post-traumatic stress disorder that went untreated following combat in their youth. The residents identified strongly with their country, their military status, and their particular branch of the service. They were all experiencing losses of health and independence related to their placement in a nursing home, and many suffered from depression and loneliness, which, in their case, was somewhat mitigated by being in an institution that supported their identity as soldiers and by being housed in barracks-type wards that prevented isolation.

The Agency Setting

My agency, my supervisor, and the members of the soldiers' home administration identified strongly with their role as caregivers for a population of veterans who had served their country. The agency, like all long-term care settings, has an insular culture and is based on a medical model of care. Because this is a state institution, bureaucracy is prevalent, and there is a focus on an administrative hierarchy, although job functions are fairly fluid. In general, there is a low turnover and strong cohesiveness among staff members. The culture of the facility values teamwork and communication, as demonstrated by a daily morning meeting in which nurse managers and support staff discuss clinical, psychosocial, administrative, and other information related to the patients and the facility. The agency is accountable to the Veterans Administration and to the Massachusetts Department of Public Health, both of which conduct annual surveys, and at the time of this evaluation was in the process of accreditation by the Joint Commission of Healthcare Organizations, a large, widely recognized independent healthcare oversight body.

Theoretical Foundations

A search of scholarly articles yielded three relevant articles that studied the benefits of participation in groups that focus on socialization of and life-review activities for the elderly. These articles led me to conclude that I should focus my evaluation on the effects of my program on the goals described above.

The first study was a commentary on considerations of clinical theory and practice related to therapeutic group interventions in the nursing home, "Group Therapy in Long-Term Care Sites," by Victor Molinari (2002). Molinari argues that because approximately half of nursing home residents have some form of dementia, a modified approach to traditional group therapy is indicated, one that pays particular attention to supporting and validating the worth of the individual. Moreover, of the "curative factors" put forth by group therapy pioneer Irving Yalom (2005), interpersonal living and group cohesion are the most relevant to the population in question due to their need to develop meaningful relationships in their new environment. Molinari, in his own review of the literature on reminiscence groups in nursing homes, indicates that up to this point there have been contradictory findings about the benefits of such groups on depression and life satisfaction. He suggests that high mortality rates in nursing homes, the lack of clarity in defining the purpose of specific interventions, and the need for the development of criteria to distinguish candidates with sufficient ego strength for intensive life reviews versus popular but less rigorous reminiscence work may be possible reasons for the ambiguity of these findings. Finally, Molinari describes the practical considerations involved in working with frail elders in such groups. These include: conducting the group at a time of the patients' maximum functioning during the day; having a more directive, flexible, and supportive therapeutic approach and being somewhat more liberal in selective self-disclosure than one might ordinarily be with other populations; and a focus on ego enhancement, rather than confrontation.

This article prompted me to clarify the purpose of my interventions by specifying in my statement of goals that it is life review, socialization, and cognitive engagement that are to be stressed in the group. I decided not to attempt to distinguish rigorously between "popular" reminiscence and "therapeutic" life review, as Molinari does, but to use my clinical judgment in providing a combination of the two to engage participants as evidenced by their affects and participation in the discussions. I also decided to follow his suggestions about providing a supportive environment at a time of day (the morning) when residents would be at their best level of functioning.

The second article, "Clinical Observations in the Treatment of World War II and Korean War Veterans with Combat-Related PTSD," by Cook, O'Donnell, Molzen, Ruzek, and Sheikh (2005), deals with a population very similar to the long-term care patients in the current events group. The authors note that older veterans have often suffered from decades of alienation and isolation. Post-traumatic stress disorder (PTSD) is actually very common in this population, with rates found in medical or inpatient psychiatric settings ranging from 9 to 80 percent. Moreover, traumatic war experiences have a detrimental effect on the health and coping of veterans, an effect that has been found to follow a waning and waxing course across their lifespan, declining in midlife and resurfacing in old age. I had observed that, in fact, many of the residents were estranged from their families, have had symptoms of psychiatric illness, and have struggled with alcohol abuse, all possible indicators for the existence of PTSD.

The empirical evidence on which this study was based on included two previous research projects for PTSD with this population. The first used group cognitive-behavioral treatment and used both the Geriatric Depression Scale (GDS; Yesavage et al., 1983) and the Impact of Events Scale (IES; Horowitz, Alvarez, & Alvarez, 1979) to measure the results. The second, which specifically addressed the symptoms of a group of veterans who were prisoners of war, used a three-stage intervention. This involved a structured discussion of events prior to military service, followed by patient education regarding trauma, and ending with an exploration of participants' concerns regarding aging, mortality, and loss. The measures used for assessment were the Symptom Checklist-90-R (SCL-90-R; Derogatis, 1992, pp. 139–45) and the Impact of Events Scale (IES; Horowitz et al., 1979). The findings in both of these projects were that improved client functioning was observed by clinicians and reported by study participants and their family members, but these results were not supported by the measures used in the studies. This would seem to suggest that the treatment was in fact beneficial and that these measures did not adequately reflect the participants' increased coping and sense of well-being.

Based on their research, Cook, O'Donnell, Molzen, Ruzek, and Sheikh developed a new model of group-therapy intervention for older veterans with PTSD. This model incorporated cognitive-behavioral interventions with educational training and a focus on coping with current stressors in a open-group treatment. The goal of the group was to decrease the veterans' symptoms of PTSD by improving their coping and sense of control. The group met weekly and focused on ongoing training about PTSD as well as the use of cognitive reframing and problem-solving techniques, learning new social skills, coping with age-related stressors, and improving family relationships. The intervention appeared to be beneficial according to the anecdotal reports of study participants and family members, as well as clinical observations, but, as in the previous studies, the instruments used to measure the outcomes did not support these results.[1] Consequently, I decided to use both measures—assessment tools and anecdotal evidence of mood and social functioning—in evaluating the benefits for my World War II and Korean War veterans.

The third study, "Research on Creativity and Aging: The Positive Impact of the Arts on Health and Illness," by Gene Cohen (2006b), had as its objective to evaluate the effects of professionally conducted cultural programs on the health and emotional well-being of elders. This was of particular interest to me because the life-review aspect of these programs was relevant to my focus on reminiscence in the current events program. The cultural programming provided under the auspices of the National Center for Creative Aging that was studied in this article was based on artistic experiences related to the participants' lives, as I knew from their literature and from participating in several of their workshops. I hoped to access some of the benefits of artistic expression based on life review that are described in this study simply through life-review activities in a group setting— in the case of the current events group, without engaging in an artistic process. My reasoning in using some of the same measures as this study to assess program results was that the current events group provided an opportunity for nursing home residents to exercise some control over their environment in making the effort to attend this optional group, which also offered an opportunity for them to develop meaningful relationships through sharing personal experiences with their peers.

In part, Cohen's study was based on gerontological research on the psychological benefits of maintaining a sense of control over some aspect of one's environment, as well as of engaging in meaningful social interactions with others. It studied elders living in the community who participated in weekly arts programming at several sites over a period of approximately two years in comparison with control groups who were on waiting lists for group participation. The Geriatric Depression Scale (Short Form), the UCLA Loneliness Scale (Russell, Cutrona, de al Mora, & Wallace, 1977), the Philadelphia Geriatric Center Morale Scale (Lawton, 1975), and various measurements of physical health and wellness yielded positive results in many areas, including gains in health and independence, social engagement, and life satisfaction. Consequently, I concluded that even without an explicit art component, a goal of the current events program could realistically be seen as promoting a sense of community among the residents and a sense of control over their lives.

II. INDICATORS OF SUCCESS

The program evaluation guidelines call for a formal statement of the criteria by which the programs can be judged a success—evidence that the objective was (or was not) accomplished. The desired outcome of the current events program is that the residents will have decreased levels of depression, increased socialization, increased coping, and fewer health declines, including decreased cognitive loss, in comparison to their counterparts who do not attend the program. This will be evidenced by patient, family, and staff reports, as well as by activity attendance records and the use of the various instruments to assess cognitive and emotional functioning.

III. DATA SOURCES

The guidelines state that the instruments that will be used as data sources are to be specified. In the case of the current events group at the soldiers' home, these were the Geriatric Depression Scale (short form), the Folstein Mini-Mental Status Exam, the UCLA Loneliness Scale, and select Minimum Data Set quality indicators of psychosocial well-being and physical functioning, including those found in Section B, Cognitive Patterns; Section C, Communicating and Understanding; Section E, Mood and Behavior Patterns; Section F, Psychosocial Well-Being; and Section N, Activity Pursuit Patterns. Moreover, HCFA Quality Indicators can be used for study purposes, including: QI 3, Prevalence of Behavioral Symptoms Affecting Others; QI 4, Prevalence of Symptoms of Depression; QI 6 Use of None or More Different Medications; QI 14, Prevalence of Weight Loss; QI 17. Incidence of Decline in Late-Loss Activities of Daily Living; and QI 23, Prevalence of Little or No Activity. I found it helpful to consult with MDS coordinators for assistance in locating this data and I urge social workers wishing to use the MDS for program evaluation purposes to do the same.

IV. EVALUATION METHODS

The guidelines call for specific information concerning evaluation methods, including who will gather the data and how it will be analyzed. As principal investigator, and with the assistance of an activity worker, I would administer the

Mini-Mental Status Exam, the Geriatric Depression Scale, and the UCLA Loneliness Scale to all residents from the old wing who proved to be eligible to participate in the current events group by report of their social worker and nurse unit manger. We would also administer a brief semistructured questionnaire to these residents, their family members (by telephone), and their nurse manager with the following questions:

1) What does the resident like best about being at the soldiers' home, and what is the most challenging thing about it?
2) What kind of choices can the resident make about how they spend their day?
3) Who is in their support network?
4) Does the resident feel that he has friends at the soldiers' home?

These questions related to some of the goals and objectives of the studies discussed in the literature review. The aim of this semistructured interview is to access some of the outcomes sought in these studies that might not necessarily be fully captured by the assessment tools, such as social engagement, sense of control, and life satisfaction.

After three months and again at six months and one year, the assessment tools and interviews would be readministered. At those times, as well, the MDS data would be reviewed for each study participant. Results for residents participating regularly in the group (that is, two to five time a week) would be studied across all assessment tools and in terms of interview reports in contrast with data on residents who do not participate regularly.

V. USE OF EVALUATION RESULTS

The final element of the evaluation framework specifies who is to receive the report on the evaluation and what use they will make of it. In this case, the evaluation results were to be presented to administration of the facility in a performance evaluation committee meeting and in a formal report. They also were to be shared with staff in a morning meeting for all nurse managers, doctors, and ancillary staff. In addition, the social service department was to discuss this report in a departmental meeting, use it to assess the quality of its current interventions, and use it to plan further programs.

As you can see from this example, having a structure for program evaluation helps to organize the process so that it seems less overwhelming to someone beginning this process and also breaks down the undertaking into a series of manageable tasks.

EVALUATION AND EVIDENCE-BASED PRACTICE

Although research has not traditionally been a part of my practice or that of most of my colleagues, evidence-based practice is a growing trend in the social work field and is here to stay. As practitioners, we cannot ignore this task because accountability is a value that both our profession and our organizational overseers are embracing. While paper compliance with this emerging mandate to engage in empirical research is an obvious concern to our profession, potentially resulting in the creation of yet more meaningless forms that we need to fill out in order to satisfy institutional funding sources, the potential benefits of seriously evaluating our clinical interventions are many. However, by more rigorously analyzing what we do that works or does not work, we are not only likely to improve our performance in terms of both efficiency and efficacy, but we will come closer to fulfilling all of the tenets of our professional mandate as embodied in the Code of Ethics of the National Association of Social Workers (1999), which states that we have a professional obligation to engage in ethically conducted research. Finally, our work is likely to earn increased legitimacy for our profession, both within our facilities and as seen by outside agencies of accreditation, thus improving the formal status of social workers in the hierarchy of our medically focused, nursing-driven work environments. In short, evaluation is power.

Of course, without prior experience, except perhaps when writing our undergraduate or master's theses, we cannot expect to acquire overnight the skills and tools we need to carry out a research-informed practice. Therefore, it is important to begin to understand this emerging phenomenon by familiarizing ourselves with the literature and taking steps to incorporate some of these techniques into our daily routines on the job. Using such a basic guideline as provided in the example above as a first step, followed by participation in professional training workshops or seminars about evidenced-based practice, as well as individual reading and discussion with colleagues, would seem to be a sensible way to build one's skills in this area.

Note

1. Instruments used to measure these outcomes included the Combat Exposure Scale (Keane et al., 1989) to verify the participants' exposure to traumatic military experiences and the PTSD Checklist–Military (Weathers, Litz, Huska, & Keane, 1993), which contains measures related to criteria for PTSD in the *Diagnostic and Statistical Manual of Mental Disorders*.

Chapter 11

Structures of Support

IN THE PREVIOUS CHAPTER ON EVALUATION, IT WAS SUGGESTED THAT social workers confer with their peers in order to master the imperative of adopting an evidence-based model of clinical practice. In fact, the process of obtaining input and support from our peers on a regular basis is crucial to our ability to remain vibrant and connected in our profession. Being an advocate is hard work. The vision for a new type of nursing home social work practice that is grounded in the concept of advocacy, specifically the idea that nursing home social workers should take an active role in shifting the paradigm of nursing home care from a medical focus to a resident-centered one, involves the social worker taking thoughtful and deliberate actions to avoid colluding with business as usual and instead seek new ways to work collaboratively with the facility on many levels to promote a focus on people and relationships.

Taking on this courageous role requires that the social worker consciously develop a support network and take any other steps necessary to ground and sustain her in her efforts. Sources of professional support can be found by joining appropriate professional committees and organizations and by finding or starting a regional support group. I'll discuss how to locate and develop these sources of support in what follows. In the long run, however, it is also important that social workers practice good self-care in order best to cope with the challenge of being a self-directed agent of change. I'll discuss that aspect of the social worker's role in what follows, as well.

"MS. FIX-IT"

Let's face it, those of us who have worked in nursing homes for any length of time know that whenever any members of the staff do not know how to handle any given situation, they call the social worker. We are accordingly asked to do any job that may be vaguely related to the residents' "psychosocial needs," which is quite a broad category, ranging from collecting overdue facility charges, to (yes) finding dentures, to asking residents to move to a different room, to addressing complex social situations that nobody else can (or wishes to) resolve. Because social workers' training provides them with a wide range of skills and because the administration and other departments at our places of employment elect to use our services as they see fit, many of us unwittingly allow our role to be defined by others. Often, it is easier to take the path of least resistance and passively to accept others' apparent assumptions, particularly if they are in authority over you, than to act decisively to carve out an independent professional identity.

GETTING THE SUPPORT WE NEED

It is too easy to internalize the dynamic tension that exists between our various responsibilities. As clinicians, we are highly attuned to the wants, needs, and emotions of others and thus at a risk from burnout due to empathy overload. Aware of the importance of support networks for our clients, we frequently as a group neglect our own mental health. However, if we consider our work situation schematically, a nursing home social worker might be depicted in her ecosystem as a solo entity, lacking emotional and professional sustenance from a varied support network. Therefore, we need to strengthen and develop the resources that we require in order to sustain ourselves in the difficult work of carrying out a professional agenda on a daily basis—an agenda that is not always recognized, appreciated, or even understood.

One major source of support is to be found in professional organizations. In what follows, I will describe the support I have received in working with other social workers both on the Massachusetts NASW Nursing Home Committee and in regional nursing home support groups. The committee has worked collectively over the past thirty years to support nursing home social workers by promoting the adoption of professional standards of practice by the NASW and the Federation of Nursing Homes, by providing an annual statewide conference for nursing home social workers, and by encouraging the formation and continued existence of informal grass-roots regional support groups by and for nursing home social workers. Regional support groups have been around even longer than the committee and provide the benefits of collegiality to nursing home social workers, who often work alone or with only a few others as auxiliary staff in nurse-managed and corporate-owned and operated settings.

The Massachusetts NASW Nursing Home Committee has made significant strides in raising the bar for the quality of social work services delivered in nursing homes. In the years before I joined the committee, the members drew up a comprehensive document entitled "Nursing Home Social Work Practice Standards." Before finalizing this document, it was reviewed and revised by numerous nursing home social workers from around the state in a variety of forums and over a period of several years. These standards were officially adopted by the NASW in 1996. Thus, the committee has had a major effect on improving the quality of social work services in long-term care settings. In addition, the committee has worked toward further implementing these standards by creating a model nursing home social work job description and by collaborating with the statewide Federation of Nursing Homes (the professional organization of nursing home administrators) to recognize facilities that adhere to the standards of practice.

Besides setting higher standards of practice for frontline social workers, for the past twenty-seven years the committee has put on an annual nursing home social work conference attracting two hundred to four hundred participants. The conference serves many purposes. It provides concrete, nuts-and-bolts information for beginning nursing home practitioners. In addition, keynote speakers discuss new developments in the care of the frail elderly, while panels and workshop leaders offer information about successful and innovative practices. Many social workers are longtime attendees and look forward to this event as the highlight of the year when they can network with their peers, share their challenges and successes, and gain inspiration that will fuel them for the year to come.

The group was originally formed to promote the enforcement of nursing home regulations implemented in the late 1960s. However, older members feel that the fledgling committee really began to jell when they organized around a crisis in the practice of nursing home social work that affected many of them directly: the threat of nursing home consultants posing as social workers without master's degrees. They brought their collective pressure to bear on this issue and, due to their efforts, the threat was eliminated. The committee continued to network and to collaborate on issues involving social change in the nursing home field. Each member brought to the table his or her own special skills and accomplishments. The members of the committee kept abreast of legislative issues, lobbied, provided testimony, and even brought nursing home residents to the statehouse to plead their case for change. Ed Alessi, in particular, through both the committee and his own organization, L.I.F.E. (Living Is For the Elderly), organized nursing home residents in grassroots groups led by his workers at nursing facilities to advocate for themselves. Due to his efforts, as well as to the political advocacy of other committee members, the state legislature passed nursing home reforms, such as the mandate for each nursing home resident in Massachusetts to have a lock box where he or she can safely store small valuables. The committee continues to be active in advocating for increases in the residents' PNA (personal needs allowance), which is money that the residents who are subsidized by the state welfare system are allowed to keep from their social security checks for their own use.

Currently, there are many opportunities for employment in the nursing home field, and the salaries for these positions are relatively high, compared with salaries in hospitals and many other settings. However, the turnover of social service directors in these facilities is high, and nursing home social work, like geriatric social work in general, continues to suffer from an ongoing lack of prestige related to the low status that society accords to the elderly. Therefore, a recent project that the committee has taken on involves networking with local schools of social work to raise students' awareness and understanding of our area of endeavor and to collaborate with colleges and universities in educating field placement supervisors and students about the nature of this work. To date, representatives from the social work education departments of two local universities have participated in brainstorming sessions with the committee to develop joint projects. One of these ideas, a competition to present a student paper at our conference, came to fruition in 2007 when a graduate student studying for a master's degree in social work presented a paper on her experience as an intern in a home-care agency placing clients in nursing homes. Additionally, the committee has made several presentations to social work students about the nature of nursing home social work as a career. In the future, both committee members and the academic field placement directors at these two schools have expressed an interest in further collaboration. We are excited about this cooperative effort because it is an opportunity for practicing workers to gain access to current theoretical thinking, as well as a way to encourage new graduates to see a nursing home job as something other than a stepping stone to a more "important" occupation.

We on the committee are convinced that our new partnership with the schools has only begun to tap what could be a potential resource for enhancing the schools' ability to provide training that is directly related to current social work practice. This training would involve the particular expectations attached to the role of nursing home social worker, as well as the development of the skills of self-advocacy in this environment.

Of the old guard, the social workers who remain are a solid group of seasoned, energetic, and enthusiastic professionals who consider themselves to be "like family" after having been privy to each other's trials and tribulations and major life changes over the years. However, the committee is very concerned about recruitment and retention of new members and works very hard to encourage younger social workers to join, to feel included in the proceedings, and to develop their own particular niche in the group. At this time, we have made it a practice for established members to "adopt" and mentor new members on an individual basis. As new members became increasingly more self-assured, they progress to taking on greater leadership roles, including that of the rotating chairmanship.

When I first began to attend the committee, I felt confused and slightly overwhelmed by the proceedings, as well by the knowledge and experience of its members. I sat in virtual silence for many months before I was ready to make a contribution, but eventually, I took on the responsibility for helping to make signs for the conference. Later, I became the committee secretary, taking notes at the meetings and sending them out to the members. My professional growth within the committee was not without setbacks. On one occasion, I submitted a paper for presentation at the annual nursing home conference that was roundly rejected, causing me deep distress at the time. Still later, I submitted a paper about a clinical experience, and it was accepted. This time, I was thrilled and excited about my success, although this brought with it an obligation to develop yet another new leadership skill, that of public speaking.

Extremely nervous, I practiced hard to prepare for this event. To my great surprise, my presentation was met with a standing ovation by the audience. This moment was pivotal in my professional development. For the first time, I felt recognized in my field and saw myself as being competent to make a worthwhile contribution to it. Eventually, I was offered and accepted the role of committee chair, a position I held for several years, and I was able to make significant contributions to the committee's mission by spearheading the effort to network with local social work schools. Now it is my turn to mentor new members, reaching out to them by phone between meetings to ensure that their needs are being met by the group.

Certainly, the pressures of family and other commitments are impediments to attending monthly meetings in the evening for the new generation of social workers. Nevertheless, I urge social workers to make such participation in a professional organization a high priority. There is strength in numbers, and it is together, not separately, that we can influence the ability of social workers to do the job that we set out to do when we graduated from social work school: to make a difference in the lives of our clients.

Joining the nursing home committee was one of the best career-related decisions I have ever made. Moreover, my experience on this committee has been invaluable in helping me to develop leadership skills. I strongly encourage everyone to join an NASW committee, in the field of aging or geriatric practice if there is no nursing home committee available in your state, so that you, too, can benefit from the support, mentorship, and opportunities for professional growth that are available.

NURSING HOME SUPPORT GROUPS

The Massachusetts NASW Nursing Home Committee has always taken an interest in keeping track of and working with nursing home social work support groups in the state of Massachusetts. At one time, these were numerous, but gradually they appear to have dwindled in number. One can only speculate about the reasons for the lack of motivation to network with our peers. However, given the fact that social workers are in the difficult position of having to advocate for our residents while being beholden to a system that often necessitates the very need for our advocacy, it is of concern that there are not more informal regional support groups in existence.

While there is some overlap in function, the NASW committee is primarily concerned with larger-scale issues and is a vehicle for advocacy for social workers, as well as for social change to benefit nursing home residents and the frail elderly in general. By contrast, a grassroots social work regional group focuses on coping with the daily stress of working on the front lines in a challenging setting. Over the years, I have had experience with a few established groups and found that they are comfortable, safe places where social workers can discuss difficult cases with their peers, exchange information about various bureaucratic forms, find out how others are dealing with particular regulations, and just relax in an atmosphere where others "speak your language," instead of being bombarded with the idiom of the medical model of nursing care.

With a colleague, Wendy, I have organized one such group and have found that the rewards of doing so are well worth the effort. Our group has gone through several transformations to accommodate our needs. In the early stages of our development, we struggled to find a common purpose and group identity. Initially, many social workers, used to working alone, could not see the benefit of meeting to discuss their jobs. In addition, we did not know each other well and lacked the trust to disclose areas of uncertainty and vulnerability. We did agree on the need for continuing professional education. Therefore, at first, we had many speakers who provided us with information about such topics as guardianship, hospice care, sexuality in the nursing home, and other relevant subjects.

In the middle stages of our group's development, we met to discuss previously agreed-upon topics such as our facilities' admission processes, in addition to holding formal training sessions with continuing education credits. In order to enhance group cohesion, we made an effort to stay on task in our discussions and to avoid digression to unrelated topics. Thus, we all had a sense that our meetings were successful in accomplishing their stated purposes.

Recently, at Wendy's behest, our meetings became much less formal. We generally convene at various restaurants for dinner each month and share what is going on with our jobs and our lives in general. The conversations include funny stories, war stories, and success stories, and we frequently ask each other for information about resources and update each other with pertinent news. (For instance, we discuss visits from the Massachusetts Department of Public Health and what they seem to be focusing on this year.) Sometimes we ask for advice about a particular case that is of concern to us. We have always been careful to maintain an agreement that specific information related to our clients is confidential, and we are careful to respect their privacy by avoiding mentioning names or other identifying information, especially when meeting in a public location. In those instances when we discuss clinical matters, the support group has functioned as a forum for peer supervision. We learn how others have handled similar situations, which provides us with both more ideas and greater confidence in handling our own work-related dilemmas.

ORGANIZING A SUPPORT GROUP

Above, I said that my friend Wendy and I organized a support group. That makes the process sound simple. As you might expect, however, the reality was a little more complicated, with the ups and downs, fits and starts, and highs and lows that characterize most worthwhile enterprises. Taking my experience as an example, here is the sort of thing you can expect when organizing a support group.

My experience with support groups began with joining an existing support group. One day at work, I got a hand-scrawled, photocopied message in the mail. Apparently, there was going to be a meeting of a local nursing home social worker support group. Feeling confused in what was still a fairly new occupation for me, I decided to attend. I hoped I could learn something from my more experienced peers. When I attended, I was not disappointed. I joined a friendly group of colleagues who were accepting, kind, and helpful at a time when I was feeling stressed, overwhelmed, and frustrated at work.

At the time, I was working in a nursing home in crisis. It was a situation in which three administrators and three directors of nursing had come and gone in the space of little over a year. As I recall, the department of public health was not overly pleased with our facility, and it seemed as though they had moved in, if not permanently, then for an extended visit. In an attempt to get a handle on the situation, the administration called meetings to address other meetings that were scheduled to resolve the original problems. These were in addition to regularly scheduled meetings, which the administration had decided to attend and to supervise, something that made me nervous. Gossip and rumors abounded. At that time, I did not have the good sense to ignore office politics and just do my job.

The support group was just that. As I shared my stories and listened to those of others, I realized that I was not alone in my situation. Some workers shared stories of similar experiences, and others offered suggestions on how to cope with various issues. Over bag lunches, coffee, and dessert, we discussed the various ways our institutions handled health department inspections, care plans, and other routines. The days that the support group met were islands of sanity in those hectic months. I owe a tremendous debt of gratitude to that group.

Then, one day, the group leader left her position, attendance suddenly dropped, and the group subsequently disbanded. Therein is the principal lesson I learned about forming and maintaining informal groups such as these: leadership is crucial. Without leadership, no one stepped up to organize the meetings, and attendance dropped. Soon, almost no one attended the meetings. Although my situation at work had improved, I still felt a great sense of loss over what I had come to count on as a part of my support network.

With the help of other social workers, I tried to resurrect the meetings, but only one or two people attended, and sometimes no one showed up for scheduled meetings. Nevertheless, I persevered. Obtaining the addresses of local nursing homes from the phone book and a publication put out by the local Federation of Nursing Homes (the administrators' organization), I sent questionnaires to local-area social workers to identify their level of interest in and their expectations for a regional group meeting, as well as which days of the week and times might be most convenient.

Quite a few social workers took the time to respond, and it turned out that they were interested in attending meetings with speakers and continuing education credits about such topics as guardianship and legal issues, advance directives such as living wills, health-care proxies, and powers of attorney, ethics, and other topics, as well as in sharing information about various policies and procedures such as admissions and discharges. Care-plan and other meetings appeared to present obstacles to attending, however, as did reluctance to leave their building during the day, both because the prospective members were busy and because of concern that their administrators would object to their absence for a few hours, monthly, to attend a professional group. However, some social workers did identify certain days of the week and times as being better than others, and from their responses, I picked the date and time that accommodated the greatest number of people. With the permission of my administrator, I held the meeting at my nursing care facility. I obtained authorization to have the food service department provide coffee and dessert for my guests. As those who are in the business of organizing meetings are undoubtedly aware, offering refreshments at the meetings is a big draw.

A few social workers arrived for the first scheduled planning meeting, among them Wendy, another social worker who had previously attended a successful regional group. Wendy expressed an interest in taking a leadership role in organizing the fledgling grassroots organization. That led to another lesson I learned about organizing such groups: you need the support of others, and when it comes to finding it, serendipity helps. Wendy and I divided up the tasks of sending out monthly invitations to the meetings, which we decided to hold at any nursing home where the social worker was interested in hosting the group.

Wendy and I also facilitated the groups. Initially and for a long time (at least a year), social workers were most likely to attend when an educational program was held. I found out that the process of having a program approved for continuing education credits involved an application to the NASW with an application fee. This fee could be recouped by charging a small amount for the training. We asked various professionals with whom we had relationships to present the programs. These included hospice workers, attorneys, and members of the Massachusetts NASW Nursing Home Committee, among others.

Over the years, the core membership of the group emerged—eight to twelve nursing home social workers, some from the same facility. All of the members started out working in close geographical proximity; over time, some members took new jobs that were farther away but still continued to attend. We are sometimes joined by the social workers who now fill their vacated positions or by others with whom we come in contact in the course of our work. As we have gotten to know each other over the years, we have developed our own traditions, such as celebrating the holidays with a special event such as a cookie exchange and taking ourselves out to a restaurant in honor of Social Work Month in March. Our level of trust has increased, and we are able both to share our concerns and to accept and value each other's assistance. We still schedule trainings with outside speakers at times, but we often meet at a restaurant in the evening with no prior agenda and feel validated and enriched by the fellowship we have created.

In the early stages of group development, we invited the facilitator of another group, a group with a great deal of longevity, to speak to us about their success. While the particulars of their meetings varied from what ours eventually became in the number of participants, frequency of meetings, and formality of the group's organization, we undertook to model ourselves closely on their strong self-advocacy. We were inspired by their tremendous pride in being nursing home social workers, by their insistence that these professional meetings were important and necessary, and by their insistence that their administrators recognize these meetings as a priority in their schedules. When one of our number was offered a directorship position at a new facility, we encouraged her to speak to her employer about her commitment to the meetings before accepting the job. As in any community, you receive support by offering it to others. But as in most communities, the leadership role played by a few individuals can be crucial.

SUPPORT YOURSELF, TOO

Because of the role that active leadership on the part of a few committed individuals plays in the organization and maintenance of informal support groups, no discussion of support is complete without mentioning the necessity to incorporate good self-care in your life, in order to be able to function at your highest level of capacity on the job, devote further energies to the group, and avoid burnout.

Those well-worn sayings about the importance of good nutrition, adequate exercise, and the practice of stress-reduction techniques such as meditation, structured relaxation, adequate sleep, journaling, and so on all are true. Each of us must find the combination of healthy practices that works best for our individual needs and lifestyles in order to be at our best at work and to have the energy to devote to the support of others in the profession. Moreover, focusing exclusively on one's career to the exclusion of one's family responsibilities and personal life is ultimately self-destructive. We must all find a balance that works for us. Finally, if continuing difficulties in one's personal or professional life become distressing, it is a good idea to seek therapy or clinical consultation around these matters.

Above all, supporting yourself means taking to heart and following the suggestions I'm articulating here for improving your role as a social worker in the nursing home system. In great part because of the unclear expectations of the social worker's position, nursing homes, like few other practice settings, provide the incredible challenge, as well as the amazing opportunity, to develop our own unique job descriptions. While this can be difficult and confusing, it is also extremely rewarding because we can use our creativity to apply the basic principles of social work in new ways to improve the lives of their residents.

THE SOCIAL WORK ROLE: A THEORETICAL PERSPECTIVE

What, in fact, is the social work role in America today? Our training teaches us some basic clinical skills for relating to our clients, skills that we refine and develop throughout our careers through interactions with clients, discussions with colleagues, and other formal and informal learning situations. We use these clinical skills to address what have been described as the three basic social work goals (Payne, 2007). The first goal is a therapeutic one: social workers assist clients in gaining understanding and control of their feelings and way of life. The second goal is transformational: social workers work to transform society to benefit the poor and oppressed. The third and last goal has to do with maintaining the status quo. In this case, social workers help individuals who have difficulties functioning to function better in order to maintain the integrity of our society. From this definition, it appears that simply doing social work–related tasks at the behest of the administration, if that is social work at all, represents a practice that is woefully focused on the maintaining a kind of social order that is in many ways detrimental to our clients and that occurs at the expense of exercising the other aspects of our professional role.

INTEGRATING PROFESSIONAL COMMITMENTS AND THE REALITIES OF PRACTICE

As I have frequently noted, a nursing home social worker is pulled in two directions by the need to comply with the corporate agenda and the mandate to use her education and skills to advocate for the frail elderly whose care has been entrusted to her. As I also have noted, the best way to maintain our social work identity in this setting and to shape a role that promotes social work goals is to be aware of this conflict, to be clear in the way we conceptualize our own job and in all of our interactions with others to serve as role models, promote our clients' emotional well-being, improve their environment, and develop community. If we do this, yes, we will still look for the occasional dentures. However, while doing so, we can consciously use the opportunity for interaction and to take a small step toward building positive alliances with staff members and clients in order to use these relationships incrementally to bring the corporate culture into better alignment with a humanistic one.

In order to reframe the practice of nursing home social work for ourselves and others, we as social workers need individually and collectively to take ownership in defining our professional role. That requires both seeking support from others and giving it in return. Being change agents can be an uphill battle and a difficult process. However, the alternative to altering the way in which we view our own position, the way in which we conduct our practice, and the way in which we present our job to others (including trainees and their schools of social work) is to risk perpetuating the problem of nursing home social workers potentially seeing themselves, being seen, and actually becoming well-meaning but somewhat hapless administrative "helpers" or (worse) agents of social control. All of this is summed up in that oft-repeated maxim articulated by Rabbi Hillel so many centuries ago: "If I am not for myself, then who will be for me? And if I am only for myself, then what am I? And if not now, when?"

Chapter 12

Final Thoughts

NOW WE HAVE COME FULL CIRCLE. IN THIS BOOK I HAVE TAKEN YOU ON A journey—the journey that began when one early career social worker began working in a long-term care institution and struggled to understand how to apply the principles of the helping profession to the world of the nursing home. I hope that my story will be of benefit to early career professionals and others who have a stake in the process of professional socialization into the field of social work As we have seen, the nursing home system is a complex one, with roots in our society's earliest attempts to deal with the "problematic" issue of caring for frail elders with limited social-support networks. Over time, specialized institutions have evolved to perform this role. The real problem here is that they do so in a stigmatizing fashion that presently has much to do with a corporate ethos of efficiency and profitability.

Currently, several grassroots organizations have formulated new ways of thinking about long-term care for the elderly, concepts much more positive than the (problem-focused) medical model that forms the basis for the present system of care. These concepts celebrate the primacy of the individual—her need to be recognized as such and to live in a community that validates her personhood. These organizations constitute a growing movement that supports the development of many innovative practices in the organizational structure and the physical environment. The grouping of residents into "neighborhoods" designed to function as mini communities, with the residents themselves directing many of their own care and lifestyle decisions, is just one of the revolutionary concepts that have been put into practice with great success in pilot programs across the country.

In a parallel way, this book advocates for reform from within existing institutions. As I have mentioned, it is of course impossible for one social worker to mandate a person-centered system of care delivery in a nursing home from her position as a minor auxiliary staff member in a medical institution. She can only use the persuasive techniques of relationship building that we have been taught to effect change one relationship at a time, building relationships with residents, staff members, and the administration based on our shared goals of helping the residents to achieve their highest level of functioning and self-actualization—although undoubtedly only a social worker would characterize it as such, and a common language needs to be developed.

This book details new uses some of the many tools for making a difference that we already have our at our disposal as trained social workers, including the ability to understand how larger systems function, to advocate, and to work with individuals and groups. Program development is one major way we can use these tools to help our clients. It has been my experience that program development is an effective, efficient way to meet the needs of a large caseload. I have described many of the programs that I have developed, as well as the process by which I put my ideas into practice. For those interested in making program development a part of your own work, I urge you to start small, with a limited objective, and build on your successes, otherwise the project is likely to become overwhelming. Always get support, both from within your institution and from outside it. You cannot effect change alone.

I have given you a system—actually, many systems, based on the social work concept of the importance of the individual. I have developed these over the years with the help of my mentors and consultants, colleagues, and residents. It is my hope that this will help you negotiate the confusing maze of conflicting agendas that characterize the worlds of our practices.

The systems that I have described for making sense of these worlds are composed of both macro and micro social work interventions. On the macro level, we can work to develop relationships with the larger elements of our organizational systems, such as the nursing department or the facility administration, treating the facility itself as a client. On the micro level, we can develop helping relationships with residents and families. As social workers, we thus need to hold multiple definitions of our clients in mind at the same time. Sometimes, it is the system, and at other times, it is the individual or small group on which we need to focus our efforts.

One of the smaller interventions comes later in the book. After talking about all of the innovative programs that we can devise, I came back to the more mundane task of completing our paperwork, but doing so in an effective way that involves understanding and visualizing each individual resident's personal information. This system can help to avoid the common pitfalls of impersonal, boilerplate care plans and care. Thus, in this way, too, we have come full circle, from learning academic concepts and clinical skills to learning to apply them in the often messy reality of the world of social work practice.

Evaluation, a concept that goes with the (not so new) reality of today's evidence-based practice is something that I have only touched upon and that constitutes a next step for me in my own professional development. The daunting need to document and justify our work suggests many new possibilities for networking with our colleagues, as well as with schools of social work, in an effort to expand the breadth and scope of our field through research.

As I have already mentioned, but cannot stress enough, networking is key. In my work, I have found it very important to have mentors, collaborators, and support in my personal life in order to do the work that I do, and I urge you to do the same. There are several types of collaboration. Some people are our natural allies; they automatically share our ideas and are enthusiastic about implementing new programs. Other collaborators are hard won and come to their work with seemingly opposing ideas of how things should be done. Both types of collaborators are important, and neither should be ignored, although it makes sense to begin to build a vital practice of program development by involving a like-minded colleague in a project of interest to both of you.

Of course, the systems I have described in this book are not a magic panacea. We all have setbacks, disappointments, conflicts, and moments of discouragement in our professional lives. At these times, step back, believe in yourself, seek support, and review in a dispassionate way the system in which you work. Know that some things are beyond your control and focus on ways to address the things that are within your control. What could you have done differently in your communication with others? What can you do now to remedy a situation that has become problematic and to build bridges to individuals and groups in the system where perhaps none existed?

Above all, it is my wish that this book be useful. As they say in AA: "Take what you want and leave the rest." Perhaps a particular program will be of interest to you, or you may find a way to start thinking about implementing one of your own devising. Whatever you chose to do, start small, build alliances, care about your individual clients, and have fun. The adventure is just beginning.

References

Abramson, J. S. (2002). Interdisciplinary team practice. In A. R. Roberts & F. J. Green (Eds.), *Social workers' desk reference* (pp. 44–50). Oxford: Oxford University Press.

Andreae, C. (2000). *When evening comes: The education of a hospice volunteer*. New York: St. Martin's Press.

Baker, B. (2007). *Old age in a new age: The promise of transformative nursing homes*. Nashville, TN: Vanderbilt University Press.

Beaulieu, E. M. (2002). *A guide for nursing home social workers*. New York: Springer Press.

Beverly Living Centers. (n.d.). *Guiding principles*. Retrieved February 8, 2008, from http://www.beverlycares.com/BL/Our+Culture/

Brock, C. 1998. *Using the senses to connect with someone who has Alzheimer's*. Excerpt from Canadian Association of Occupational Therapists & Alzheimer Society of Canada, Living at home with Alzheimer's disease and related dementias: A manual of resources, references and information. Ottawa, ON: CAOT Publications. Retrieved February 17, 2008, from www.OTworks.ca

Brody, E. (1974). *A social work guide for long-term care facilities*. Rockville, MD: National Institute of Mental Health.

Brun, C. F. (2005). *A practical guide to social service evaluation*. Chicago: Lyceum Books.

Butler, R. (1963). The life review: An interpretation of reminiscence in the aged. *Psychiatry, 26*(1), 65–76.

Calderon, K. S. (2001). Making the connection between depression and activity levels among the oldest-old: A measure of life satisfaction. *Activities, Adaptation, and Aging, 25*(2), 59.

Cohen, G. (2001). *The creative age: Awakening human potential in the second half of life* New York: HarperCollins.

Cohen, G. (2006a). *The mature mind: The positive power of the aging brain*. New York: Basic Books.

Cohen, G. (2006b). Research on creativity and aging: The positive impact of the arts on health and illness. *Generations, 30*(1), 7–15.

Cook, J., O'Donnell, C., Molzen, J., Ruzek, J., & Sheikh, J. (2005). Clinical observations in the treatment of World War II and Korean War veterans with combat-related PTSD. *Clinical Gerontologist, 29*(2), 83–84.

Coste, J. K. (2003). *Learning to speak Alzheimer's: A groundbreaking approach for everyone dealing with the disease*. Boston: Houghton Mifflin.

Derogatis, L. R. (1992). *SCL-90-R: Administration, scoring and procedure, manual-II*. Townsend, MD: Clinical Psychometric Research.

Devanand, D. P., et al. (2000). Olfactory deficits in patients with mild cognitive impairment predict Alzheimer's Disease at follow-up. *American Journal of Psychiatry 157* (September), 1399–1404

Downton, E. (2007, May). *The other side of the bedpan*. Paper presented at the National Association of Social Workers Nursing Home Committee conference in Bedford, MA.

Dreeszen, C. (2003). *Fundamentals of arts management.* Amherst: Arts Extension Service, Division of Continuing Education, University of Massachusetts.

Duhigg, C. (2007, September 23). At many homes, more profit and less nursing. *New York Times.*

Erikson, E. H., Erikson, J. M., & Kivnick, H. Q. (1987). *Vital Involvement in Old Age.* New York: W. W. Norton and Co.

Fagan, R. M. (2003). Changing the culture of aging in America. In A. S. Weiner & J. L. Ronch (Eds.), *Culture change in long-term care* (pp. ???). New York: Haworth Social Work Practice Press. 134.

Fischer, J. (1978). *Effective casework practice.* New York: McGraw Hill.

Gabriel, C. S. (2000). *An overview of nursing home facilities: Data from the 1997 National Nursing Home Survey.* Advance Data No. 311. Hyattsville, MD: National Center for Health Statistics, Retrieved May 14, 2008, from http://www.cdc.gov/nchs/products/pubs/pubd/ad/311-320/ad311.htm

Genesis Healthcare. (n.d.). *Vision.* Retrieved February 8, 2008, from http://www.genesishcc.com/index.cfm?page_id=35

Gibson, F. (2004). *The past in the present: Using reminiscence in health and social care.* Baltimore, MD: Health Professions Press.

Gigliotti, Christine M., et al. (2004). Harvesting health: effects of three types of horticultural therapy activities for persons with dementia. *Dementia, 3*(2), 173.

Goffman, E. (1961). *Asylums: Essays on the social situation of mental patients and other inmates.* Garden City, NY: Doubleday Anchor Books.

Hammond, D. (2003). *The science of synthesis: Exploring the social implications of general systems theory.* Boulder: University of Colorado Press.

Harrington, C., Carrillo, H., & Woleslagle Blank, B. (September, 2007). *Nursing facilities, staffing, residents and facility deficiencies, 2000 through 2006.* San Francisco: Department of Social and Behavioral Sciences, University of California. Retrieved February 23, 2009 from http://www.nccnhr.org/uploads/HarringtonOSCARcomplete2006.pdf

Horowitz, M., Alvarez, N., & Alvarez, W. (1979.) The Impact Event Scale: A measure of subjective stress. *Psychosomatic Medicine, 41*(3), 209–18.

Kaffenberger, K. R. (2001). Nursing home ownership: An historical analysis. *Journal of Aging and Social Policy, 12*(1), 35.

Keane, T. M., Fairbank, J. A., Aimering, R. T., Taylor, K. L, et al. (1989). Clinical evaluation of a measure to assess combat exposure. *Psychological Assessment, 1*(1), 53–55.

Lawton, M. P. (1975). The Philadelphia Geriatric Center Morale Scale: A revision. *Journal of Gerontology, 30*(1), 85–89.

Lévi-Strauss, C. (1966). *The savage mind.* Chicago: University of Chicago Press.

Lichtenberg, J. D. (1975). The development of a sense of self. *Journal of the American Psychological Association, 23,* 453–461.

Loss of smell linked to key protein in Alzheimer's Disease. *Science Daily,* Philadelphia, PA, March 12, 2004.

McLean, A. (1997). *The person in dementia: A study of nursing home care in the U.S.* (Orchard Park, NY: Broadview Press.

McLean, A. (2007). *The person in dementia: A study of nursing home care in the US.* Peterborough, ONT: Broadview Press, 224–45.

Molinari, V. (2002). Group therapy in long-term care sites. *Clinical Gerontologist, 25*(1–2), 13–24.

National Association of Social Workers. (1999). *Code of ethics of the National Association of Social Workers.* Retrieved February 8, 2008, from http://www.socialworkers.org/pubs/code/code.asp

National Association of Social Workers, Massachusetts Chapter. (1996). *Nursing Home Social Work Practice Standards.* Retrieved February 23, 2009, from http://old.naswma.org/join/default.asp?contentID=343&topicID=98

Newman, K. (1984). The capacity to use the object. In G. H. Pollock & J. E. Gedo (Eds.), *Clinical psychoanalysis and its applications* (pp. ???). New York: International Universities Presses.

Payne, M. (2007). *What is professional social work?* (2nd ed.). Chicago: Lyceum Books.

Pelland, R. (2000). *Creativity in the nursing home.* Workshop at the Massachusetts National Association of Social Workers Nursing Home Conference, Waltham, MA.

Polikoff, B. G. (1999). *With one bold act: The story of Jane Addams.* Chicago: Boswell Books.

Rothman, D. (1971). *The discovery of the asylum: Social order and disorder in the new republic.* Glenview, IL: Scott, Foresman.

Rubenstein, N. (2005). Psychic homelands and the imagination of place: A literary perspective. In G. Rowles & H. Chaudhury (Eds.), *Home and identity in late life: International perspectives* (pp. 111–36). New York: Springer.

Russell, D. W., Cutrona, C. E., de al Mora, A., & Wallace, R. B. (1977). Loneliness and nursing home admission among the rural elderly. *Psychology and Aging, 12*, 574–89.

Schafer, D. (1994). *Reminiscing and nursing home life.* London: Garland.

Sheikh, J. I., & Yesavage, J. A. (1986). Geriatric Depression Scale: Recent evidence and development of a shorter version. *Clinical Gerontolology, 5,* 165–172.

Shield, R. R. (1988). *Uneasy endings: Daily life in an American nursing home.* Ithaca, NY: Cornell University Press.

Stafford, P. B. (Ed.). (2003). *Gray areas: Ethnographic encounters with nursing home culture.* Santa Fe, NM: School of American Research Press.

Stricker, G., & Gold, J. R. (1988). A psychodynamic approach to the personality disorders. *Journal of Personality Disorders, 2*(4), 350–359.

Suggs, P., & Suggs, D. (2003). The understanding and creation of rituals: Enhancing the life of older adults. *Journal of Religious Gerontology, 15*(3), 17–18.

Sun Healthcare Corporation. (n.d.). *See what's new under the sun.* Retrieved February 8, 2008, from http://www.sunh.com/Production/AboutSHG/sun_mission_values.asp

Tharp, T. (2003). *The creative habit: Learn it and use it for life. A practical guide* (New York: Simon and Schuster.

Tobin, S. (2003). The historical context of "humanistic" culture change in long-term care. In A. S. Weiner & J. L. Ronch (Eds.), *Culture change in long-term care* (pp. ???). New York: Haworth Social Work Practice Press. 54.

Trattner, W. (1994). *From poor law to welfare state: A history of social welfare in America* (6th ed.). New York: Free Press. 80.

van der Hart, O. (1983). *Rituals in psychotherapy: Transition and continuity.* (A. Pleit-Kuiper, Trans.). New York: Irvington.

van Gennep, A. (1960). *The rites of passage.* Chicago: University of Chicago Press.

Voelkl, J. E. (1985). Effects of institutionalization upon residents of extended care facilities. *Activities, Adaptation & Aging,* 3/4, 37–45.

Weathers, F., Litz, B., Huska, J., & Keane, T. (1993, October). *The PTSD Checklist (PCL) Reliability, Validity and Diagnostic Utility.* Paper presented at the Annual Convention of the International Society for Traumatic Stress Studies, San Antonio, TX.

Weiner, J. M., Freiman, M. P., Brown, D., & RTI International. (2007, December). *Nursing home care quality twenty years after the Omnibus Budget Reconciliation Act of 1987.* A Kaiser Family Foundation Report. Retrieved February 8, 2008, from http://www.kff.org/medicare/upload/7717.pdf

Woodruff, K. (1971). *From charity to social work in England and the United States.* Toronto: University of Toronto Press.

Wiersma, E. (2000). Institutionalization of seniors: A necessary practice? *Journal of Leisurablity, 27*(1) Retrieved February 18, 2008, from http://adp.lin.ca/resource//html/Vol27/V27N1A4.htm

Wolinsky, F. D., Callahan, C. M., Fitzgerald, J. F., & Johnson, R. J. (1992). The risk of nursing home placement and subsequent death among older adults. *Journal of Gerontolology, 47*(4), S173–182.

Wunderlich, G. S., & Kohler, P. O. (Eds.) (2001). *Improving the quality of long-term care.* Washington, DC: National Academy Press.

Yalom, I. (2005). *Theory and practice of group psychotherapy.* New York: Basic Books.

Yan, M. C. (2008). Exploring cultural tensions in cross-cultural social work. *Social Work, 53*(4), 317–328.

Yeatts, D. E., & Cready, C. M. (2007). The consequences of empowered CNA teams in nursing home settings: A longitudinal assessment. *Gerontologist, 47,* 323–339.

Yesavage, J. A., Brink, T. L., Rose, T. L., Lum, O., Huang, V., Adey, M. B., & Leirer, V. O. (1983). Development and validation of a geriatric depression rating scale: A preliminary report. *Journal of Psychological Research, 17*(27), 37–49.

Zauszniewski, J. A., et al. (2004). Focused reflection reminiscence group for elders. *Journal of Applied Gerontology, 23*(4), 429–442.

Index

About the Author

JULIE SAHLINS WAS BORN IN NEW YORK, AND RAISED MOSTLY IN ANN Arbor, Michigan with family trips to California, the Pacific Islands, and France. She attended Smith College and graduated from Boston University with a BFA in painting. This was followed by an MFA in art education. Some years later Julie earned her MSW at Simmons College. Since that time she has worked primarily with the elderly in a variety of nursing home settings. She is clinical social worker at the Chelsea Soldiers' Home. Julie enjoys volunteering in the community and has recently returned to her art. She lives in Newton, Massachusetts with her two feline assistants.